Extending P

Mike Reiners
7/10/03

EXTENDING PRACTICAL MEDICINE

Fundamental Principles based on the Science of the Spirit

RUDOLF STEINER, PhD
and
ITA WEGMAN, MD

Translated by A.R. Meuss, FIL, MTA

RUDOLF STEINER PRESS
London

Rudolf Steiner Press
51 Queen Caroline Street
London W6 9QL

www.rudolfsteinerpress.com

Previously published in English as *Fundamentals of Therapy*
First edition 1925, Anthroposophical Publishing Co., London
Second edition 1938, Anthroposophic Press, New York
Third edition 1967 and fourth edition 1983, Rudolf Steiner Press, London
This edition 1996
Reprinted 2000

Originally published in German under the title *Grundlegendes für eine
Erweiterung der Heilkunst nach geisteswissenschaflichen Erkenntnissen*
(volume 27 in the *Rudolf Steiner Gesamtausgabe* or Collected Works) by
Rudolf Steiner Verlag, Dornach. This authorized translation published by
kind permission of the Rudolf Steiner Nachlassverwaltung, Dornach

Translation © Rudolf Steiner Press 1996

A catalogue record for this book is available from the British Library

ISBN 1 85584 080 4

Cover by Andrew Morgan
Typeset by DP Photosetting, Aylesbury, Bucks
Printed and bound in Great Britain by Cromwell Press Limited

Contents

Foreword

In this book Rudolf Steiner and Ita Wegman lay a foundation for a future medicine that can do justice to the human being as a being of spirit and soul and not merely as a physical object. Although modern medical science has vastly increased our understanding of the human body and given us many powerful life-saving techniques, its methods of study are essentially no different from the methods of study of other physical objects in the world. In this book, Rudolf Steiner and Ita Wegman point to a path of training and a research method, no less exacting than the scientific method, which can yield knowledge of a quite different nature about the phenomenon of life, the soul and spirit. Such knowledge can bear fruit in the practice of medicine.

Before the advent of science, the human being was known to be part of a universe experienced as spiritual, as well as physical in nature. For many centuries such teachings relied on the authority of the past, but there are also indications that in the more distant past such knowledge could be acquired directly within the confines of ancient 'mystery' centres. Here the pupil to be initiated was led, after a long preparation, to a direct experience of spiritual realities. The authors do not advocate the return to a pre-scientific consciousness or to some kind of religious belief system. Rather, theirs is the intention to build on what science has brought to humanity, and on this basis, reopen the path of initiation appropriate to the human beings of the twentieth and subsequent centuries.

In addition to its content, the way in which this book came about holds keys for the future development of a spiritualised medicine of the future. The book is unique as it is the only written work, as opposed to lectures, that Rudolf Steiner published on a professional sphere of work. It is also the only book which he wrote together with another author. The opening chapters of the book have a certain directness and straightforwardness, others pose substantial challenges to comprehension. It is a book to live with, and come back to, rather than a book containing information which can be rapidly assimilated and put into practice.

The central theme in the anthroposophical under-standing both of the human body and world of sub-stances which surrounds us is the need to see the substances in terms of their process of formation, rather than seeing them as 'things'. It is revealing also to look at this book itself in terms of the process which created it, and in terms of the processes which it can, in turn, inspire. The chapters came about in conversations between Rudolf Steiner and Ita Wegman in which he described to her the main ideas for each particular chapter. However, they were only written down later by Ita Wegman after she had slept on these ideas. She then returned her written expression of them to Rudolf Stei-ner, who amended them to create the final manuscript.

This rather unusual process sounds like an echo of what Rudolf Steiner describes of the kinds of conversa-tion that took place between the initiate and the pupil in the mysteries of Ephesus (in lectures given in August 1924 in Torquay, England). There, he describes how, while walking through the groves surrounding the

Temple, the initiate/teacher would describe the plants' 'connection' to specific influences in the cosmos. Then, at night, the pupil would experience in sleep the related life processes present both within the plant and the human organism, and relate these to the teacher in following conversations. What the pupil would bring as a response from sleep would complement and complete the wisdom that the teacher-initiate could bring. Through this process involving two individuals, a form of spiritual wisdom related both to the cosmos and its earthly reflection in physiological processes could be researched. The writing of this book appears to be a modern-day equivalent of such a process of the ancient mysteries.

In the same cycle of lectures, Rudolf Steiner indicates that to research spiritual knowledge of physiology, for example the spiritual physiology of the human organs, requires more than one individual advanced initiate, in order to anchor and express such spiritual perceptions. We have here an indication that if the medicine of the future is to be spiritually inspired, its research will be a co-operative venture of groups of individuals. The development of case conferences in anthroposophical medical centres and groups doing research into medicinal substances is perhaps a beginning of working in this spirit. When such activity takes its beginning from this book, then the conversation which brought this book into being is finding its continuation.

Dr Michael Evans
Michaelmas 1996
Stroud, Glos.

1
Understanding the True Nature of Man as a Basis of Medical Practice

This small book presents new approaches in medical knowledge and skills. A proper judgement of its contents will only be possible for those who are prepared to consider the points of view that were dominant when the medical views discussed in these pages evolved.

It is not a matter of being in opposition to the school of medicine that is working with the accepted scientific methods of the present time. We fully acknowledge its principles. And in our view, the approach we present should only be used by those who are fully able and entitled to practise medicine according to those principles.

We do, however, add further insights to such knowledge of the human being as is now available through accepted scientific methods. These are gained by different methods, and we therefore feel compelled to work for an extension of clinical medicine, based on these *wider* insights into the nature of the world and the human being.

Basically those who follow the established practice of medicine cannot object to what we are presenting because we do not go against that practice. The only people who can refuse to accept our attempt without further ado are those who not only demand that we accept their system of knowledge but also insist that no insights may be presented that go beyond their system.

Extended insight into the nature of the world and the human being is in our view offered in anthroposophy, an approach established by Rudolf Steiner. To our understanding of the *physical* human being, which can only be gained by the methods of natural science,* it adds understanding of the *non-physical* or *spiritual* human being. Anthroposophy does not involve progressing from insight into the physical to insight into the spiritual aspect by merely thinking about it. This would only produce more or less well thought-out hypotheses, with no one able to prove that they are in accord with reality.

Before anything is said in anthroposophy about the spiritual aspect, methods are developed that entitle one to make such statements. To get some idea of these methods, readers are asked to consider the following. All findings made in established modern science are essentially based on impressions gained through the human senses. Human beings may extend their ability to perceive what the senses can provide by means of experiments or through observations made using instruments, but this adds nothing *essentially* new to knowledge gained in that world in which human beings live through their senses.

Thinking, in so far as it is applied to investigating the physical world, also does not add anything to the evidence of our senses. In thinking we combine, analyse, etc. sensory impressions to arrive at laws (of nature); those who investigate the world of the senses must, however,

---

* 'Natural science' (or 'modern science'), which nowadays is generally referred to just as 'science', is here given its original name to avoid confusion with 'spiritual science' or 'the science of the spirit'. Translator.

say to themselves: the thinking which thus wells up in me does not add anything real to the reality of the world perceived by the senses.

This will change as soon as human beings do not limit themselves to the level of thinking that they initially develop through life, upbringing and education. We can strengthen our thinking and increase its power. We can focus the mind on simple, limited thoughts and then, excluding all other thoughts, concentrate the whole power of soul on such ideas. A muscle gains in strength if tensed repeatedly, the forces always being in the same direction. Inner powers of soul are strengthened in the sphere that normally governs thinking by doing exercises of the kind just mentioned. It has to be emphasized that the exercises must be based on simple, limited thoughts. For the soul should not be exposed to influences that are half or even fully unconscious during those exercises. (Only the principle of the exercises can be given here; for full details and directions on how to do such exercises, see Rudolf Steiner's *Knowledge of the Higher Worlds, Occult Science*, and other anthroposophical writings.[1])

The most obvious objection to this is that if the whole power of soul is directed to a specific thought, focusing on it completely, all kinds of autosuggestion and the like may arise, and one simply begins to imagine things. It is, however, also shown in anthroposophy how the exercises should go, so that the objection is null and void. It is shown that in doing the exercises one proceeds in full presence of mind just as one does in solving a problem in arithmetic or geometry. The mind cannot lapse into unconscious spheres when solving such problems, nor can it do so if the directions given in anthroposophy are carefully followed.

Doing the exercises strengthens the *powers of thought* to a previously undreamt-of degree. We feel powers of thought active in us like a new content in the essence of our being. And as our own being is given new content, the world, too, is perceived to have a content of which we may have had a vague idea before but which we have not known from experience. Considering our ordinary thinking in moments of self-observation, we find our thoughts to be shadow-like and pale compared to the impressions gained through the senses.

Perceptions gained through enhanced powers of thinking are far from pale and shadowy; they are full of content, utterly real images; their reality is much more intense than is found in the content of our sensory impressions. A new world opens up for human beings when they have extended their powers of perception in the indicated way.

Learning to have perceptions in this world where before they were only able to have perceptions in the world of the senses, people realize that all the laws of nature they knew before apply *only* in the physical world; and that the nature of the world they have now entered is such that its laws are different, indeed the opposite of those in the physical world. In this world, the law of the earth's force of attraction does not apply, but rather the opposite, for a force presents itself that does not act outwards from the centre of the earth but the other way round, from the periphery of the universe to the centre of the earth. And the same holds true for the other forces of the physical world.

In anthroposophy, the ability to perceive this world gained through exercises is called the power of imaginative perception. Imaginative not because one is dealing with 'figments of the imagination' but because the contents of the conscious mind are not thought shadows but images. Sensory perception gives direct experience of being in a real world, and so does the inner activity of gaining imaginative knowledge. The world to which this perception relates is called the etheric world in anthroposophy. This is not the hypothetical ether of modern physics, but something truly perceived in the spirit. The name is used because it relates to earlier, instinctive ideas of this world. Compared to the clear perceptions now possible these ideas no longer have validity; but we have to give names to things if we wish to refer to them.

Within this ether world it is possible to perceive an etheric bodily nature that exists in addition to the physical bodily nature of the human being.

Our etheric bodily nature is something that in essence exists also in the plant world. Plants have an ether body. The laws of physics actually apply only in the world of lifeless minerals.

The plant world is possible on earth because there are substances in the earth-sphere that are not limited to the laws of physics but may leave all physical laws behind and adopt laws that go in the opposite direction. The laws of physics act as though streaming out from the earth; etheric laws act as though streaming to the earth from all sides of the world periphery. We can only understand the developing plant world if we see how in it earthly physical principles interact with etheric and cosmic principles.

And that is how it is with regard to the human etheric body. Because of it, something happens in the human being that is not a continuation of forces of the physical body acting according to their laws, but happens because physical substances rid themselves of their physical forces as soon as they stream into the etheric.

At the beginning of a human life on earth—most clearly so during the embryonic period—the forces of the etheric body act as powers of configuration and growth. As life progresses, a part of these forces becomes emancipated from activity in configuration and growth and is transformed into powers of thought, the very powers that create the shadowy thought world we have in ordinary consciousness.

It is of the greatest importance to know that ordinary human powers of thought are refined powers of configuration and growth. A spiritual principle reveals itself in the configuration and growth of the human organism. And as life progresses this principle emerges as the spiritual power of thought.

And this power of thought is only one part of the power of human configuration and growth that is at work in the etheric. The other part remains faithful to the function it had at the beginning of human life. Human beings continue to develop when configuration and growth have reached an advanced stage, that is, to some degree a conclusion, and it is because of this that the non-physical, spiritual etheric which is alive and actively at work in the organism is able to become power of thought in later life.

The power to change and be changed thus presents itself to imaginative perception in one aspect as being etheric and spiritual and in its other aspect as the soul content of thinking.

If we consider the substantial nature of earthly substances and follow how they are worked on by the etheric, we have to say: wherever the substances enter into this creative process, they develop an essential nature that estranges them from physical nature. Becoming estranged, they enter into a world where the spiritual principle meets them and transforms them so that they assume its own nature.

To rise to the living, etheric nature of the human being in the way described here is something utterly different from the unscientific insistence on a 'vital force' that was commonly used in the attempt to explain living bodies up to the middle of the nineteenth century. Here it is a matter of directly perceiving—in mind and spirit—an essential principle that exists in humans and all other life forms just as the physical body does. To gain this perception we do not continue the ordinary way of thinking in some vague fashion, nor do we make up another world using our powers of fantasy. Instead, human perceptiveness is extended in a highly specific way, and this then also leads to experience of a wider world.

The exercises that lead to higher perception may be taken further. Having made an extra effort to concentrate on specific thoughts, it is also possible to make an extra effort to suppress the imaginations (images of a spiritual, etheric reality) that have been achieved. The resulting state is a completely empty conscious mind. One is merely awake, and this waking state initially has no content. (Details are given in the above-mentioned books.) This waking state without content does not continue, however. Having been emptied of all physical and all image-like etheric impressions it fills with a content that streams to it from a real world of the spirit, just as impressions gained of the physical world stream towards the physical senses.

Through imaginative perception we got to know a

second aspect of our human nature; when the empty conscious mind fills with spiritual content we get to know a third aspect. In anthroposophy, perceptive insight arrived at in this way is said to come through Inspiration. (These terms should not put the reader off; they have been taken from an instinctive way of seeing worlds of spirit that belongs to primitive times; their meaning in the present context is exactly stated.) The world to which we gain access through Inspiration is called the astral world in anthroposophy.—Speaking of an etheric world in the terms used in these pages, we refer to the influences that take effect from the world periphery in the direction of the earth. Speaking of an 'astral world', however, we progress, in accord with what the inspired conscious mind observes, from influences coming from the world periphery to specific spirit entities who are revealed in those influences, just as the physical substances of the earth reveal their nature in the forces emanating from the earth. We speak of distinct spirit entities acting from the far distances of the universe just as we speak of stars and constellations when we use the senses to look at the night sky. Hence the term 'astral world'. In this astral world human beings have the third aspect of their essential nature: the astral body.

Earthly substantiality must also stream into this astral body. In the process it becomes further estranged from its physical nature.—Human beings thus have their ether body in common with the plant world and their astral body with the animal world.

The essentially human element that raises humanity above the animal world is perceived and becomes known through a form of perceptive insight that is even higher than Inspiration. This is called 'Intuition' in anthroposophy. In Inspiration, a world of spiritual entities reveals itself; in Intuition, the relationship of the perceptive human being to this world becomes a closer one. Something purely spiritual is brought to full conscious awareness, and conscious experience of this immediately shows that this has nothing to do with experience gained in our bodily nature. We thus enter into a life where we are human spirit among other spiritual entities. In Inspiration, the spiritual entities of the world *reveal* themselves; through Intuition we *live* with those spirits.

We thus come to recognize the fourth aspect of essential human nature, the 'I' itself. Again we become aware that in making itself part of the essence and active working of the 'I', earthly substantiality becomes even further estranged from its physical nature. The essential nature this substantiality assumes as 'I organization' is initially the form in which earthly matter is most estranged from the physical nature it has on Earth.

The 'astral body' and 'I' we thus encounter are not tied to the physical body in the human organization the way the etheric body is. Inspiration and Intuition show that 'astral body' and 'I' separate from physical and etheric body during sleep, and that complete interpenetration of the four aspects of human nature to create an integral human entity exists only in the waking state.

In sleep, the physical and etheric human body remain in the physical and etheric world. They are not, however, in the position in which the physical and etheric body of a plant are. They hold the after-effects of the astral and I principles. And the moment they would no longer hold these after-effects the individual must wake up. A human physical body must never be left merely to physical, a human ether body never merely to etheric influences. They would then disintegrate.

Inspiration and Intuition also show something else, however. Physical substantiality knows further development of its essential nature when it proceeds to be alive and actively working in the etheric. And *life* depends on the organic body being torn away from earthly nature and built up from the universe that lies beyond the earth. Such constructive development only results in *life*, however, and not in *conscious awareness* nor in *self awareness*. The astral body needs to build its organization within the physical and etheric organization; the I needs to do the same with regard to the I organization. Yet this *building-up process* does not lead to conscious development of an inner life of soul. For this to happen, constructive development has to be countered with *destruction*. The astral body builds its organs; it breaks them down again by letting the activity of feeling develop in the soul's inner awareness; the I evolves its 'I organization'; it breaks it down again as will activity takes effect in self awareness.

The spirit does *not* develop on the basis of *constructive* but of *destructive* activity of matter in the essential human being. If spirit is to be active in man, matter must withdraw from this activity.

Even the development of thinking activity within the etheric body is not based on a continuation of etheric nature but on its destruction. *Conscious* thinking does *not* take place in processes of configuration and growth, but in processes of defiguration and withering, dying, which are continually integrated into the etheric process.

In conscious thinking, thoughts come free of the

physical configuration process and as soul configurations become living human experiences.

If we consider the human being on the basis of this approach to human nature, we realize that it is only possible to get full insight into both the human being as a whole and into an individual organ if we know how the physical body, the etheric body, the astral body and the I are active in them. In some organs the I is predominantly active; in others the I shows little activity, and the physical organization predominates.

We can only fully understand the healthy human being if we know how the higher aspects of human nature take hold of earthly substance and compel it to serve them, and if we also realize that earthly substance changes when it enters into the sphere of activity of the higher aspects of human nature; in the same way we can only understand the sick human being if we realize the situation which arises for the organism as a whole, for an organ or a sequence of organs if the higher aspects' mode of action becomes irregular. And we shall only be able to think of medicines when we develop knowledge of how an earthly substance or earthly process relates to the etheric, to the astral, to the I. Only then will it be possible to introduce an earthly substance into the human organism or to treat the organism with an earthly activity to such effect that the higher aspects of the human being are able to develop unhindered, or, of course, that earthly substantiality gains the support it needs from what has been added to it, so it may go in a direction where it becomes the foundation for the work of the spirit on Earth.

Man is what he is through physical body, ether body, soul (astral body) and I (spirit). In health human beings must be considered in terms of these aspects, in sickness perceived in terms of the balance between them being upset; for health, it is necessary to find medicines that will restore the upset balance.

An approach to medicine based on these foundations is outlined in this book.

2
Why Do People Fall Ill?

Anyone taking the modern scientific approach gets caught up in contradiction when reflecting on the fact that people may be ill, and initially has to assume this contradiction to be due to the nature of existence as such. At first sight, a disease is a natural process. Yet the process that takes its place in health is equally natural.

Natural processes are known primarily from observation of the world outside the human being, and from observation of the human being only in so far as this is done in exactly the same way as observation of nature, outside. The human being is seen as a part of nature which is such that the processes that can also be observed outside are highly complex in this part of nature yet are nevertheless of the same kind as those in outside nature.

But this is where a question arises that cannot be answered from this point of view. How do natural processes develop in the human being—leaving animals aside for the moment—that are the opposite of healthy processes?

The healthy human organism seems comprehensible as part of the natural world; the diseased organism does not seem to be such. It must therefore be comprehensible on its own terms, through something it does not have from the natural world.

The idea seems to be that the spiritual, non-physical aspect of the human being has a complex natural process as its physical basis, which is like a continuation of the natural principles that pertain outside the human being. But simply consider—will continuation of a natural process based on a healthy human organism ever bring the mind and spirit alive? The opposite is the case. The life of mind and spirit is extinguished if the natural process continues in a straight line. This happens in sleep; it happens in a faint.

Consider on the other hand how the conscious life of mind and spirit becomes more acute when an organ is diseased. Pain develops, or at least a reluctance to do things or discomfort. The life of feeling gains a content it does not otherwise have. And the life of the will is impaired. The movement of a limb, which happens as a matter of course in health, cannot be performed because pain or reluctance inhibit it.

Observe the transition from painful movement of a limb to its paralysis. Pain on movement marks the first step towards paralysis. The active spiritual principle intervenes in the organism. In health it initially reveals itself in the life of ideas, of thought. We activate an idea; and the movement of a limb follows. We do not enter consciously with our idea into the organic processes that ultimately lead to movement of the limb. The idea goes down to the unconscious level. In health, a feeling process develops between idea and movement that is active only at soul level. It does not distinctly connect with anything physical and organic. In ill health this does happen, however. Feeling, which in health is experienced as separate from the physical organism, connects with it in the experience of illness.

The processes of healthy feeling and disease-related experience are thus seen to be related. There has to be something which in a healthy organism is not connected as intensely with that organism as in a sick organism. This reveals itself to spiritual perception as the astral body. It is an organization beyond sensory perception that lies within the sense-perceptible organization. It either intervenes loosely in an organ, which leads to inner soul experience that exists on its own and is not felt to be connected with the body, or it intervenes intensely in an organ; this leads to the experience of illness. We have to develop the idea of one form of illness where the astral body takes hold of the organism, which makes the spiritual human being enter more deeply into his body than is the case in health.

However, thinking also has its physical basis in the organism. It is only that in health it is even more detached from the organism than feeling is. Spiritual perception finds that in addition to the astral body there is a separate I organization which lives as an independent soul quality in our thinking. If the human being enters intensely into the bodily aspect with this I organization, a condition arises in which observation of one's own organism is similar to that of the outside world.—If we observe an object or event in the outside world, the fact is that the thought in the human mind and the object or event observed are not in live interaction but independent of each other. This only happens with a human limb if it becomes paralysed. It then becomes outside world. The I organization is no longer loosely connected with the limb the way it is in health, when it can connect with the limb in a movement and immediately let go again; it enters permanently into the limb and can no longer withdraw.

Again we have the healthy movement processes of a limb in juxtaposition with paralysis and see how they relate. Indeed, we can see quite clearly that a healthy movement is the beginning of a paralysis that is cancelled as soon as it begins.

We have to consider the nature of illness to lie in an intense connection of the astral body or I organization with the physical organism. But this connection is merely an enhancement of the looser connection that exists in a state of health. Thus even the normal interventions of astral body and I organization in the human body relate not to healthy vital processes but to pathological ones. When spirit and soul take effect, they cancel out the normal way the body is constituted; they change it into its opposite. With this, however, they put the organism on a road where illness wants to begin. In ordinary life this is regulated as soon as it arises by a self-healing process.

A certain form of illness develops if the spiritual or soul aspect advance too far towards the organism, so that self-healing will either not come about at all or only do so slowly.

The causes of illness must thus be sought in the capacity for spirit and soul. And healing must consist in releasing the soul or spirit element from the physical organization.

This is one form of illness. There is also another. The I organization and the astral body may be prevented from establishing the loose connections with the bodily aspect that in ordinary existence are the basis of independent feeling, thinking and will. Healthy processes then go beyond the level that is appropriate for the organism in the organs or processes that cannot be reached by spirit and soul. And in this case spiritual perception shows that the physical organism will then do more than merely perform the lifeless processes of outside nature. The physical organism is penetrated by an etheric organism. On its own, the physical organism could never evoke a self-healing process. This is fanned into life in the etheric organism. With this we realize that health is a condition that has its origin in the etheric organism. Healing must thus consist in treating the etheric organism.*

---

* A comparison of what has been said in the first chapter with the contents of the second chapter will specifically help the reader understand the point at issue.

3
The Phenomena of Life

Understanding of the healthy and sick human organism will not be gained if we imagine that the activity of some substance taken in with the food simply continues to act in the inner organism the way it did in outside nature. It is not a matter of the activity we observe the substance to have outside the human organism continuing on, but of it being overcome.

The mistaken notion that substances from the outside world continue to act in their specific way inside the organism arises because that seems to be the case if one thinks in the way people usually do in chemistry. Having done their investigations they believe that hydrogen, for instance, is the same in the organism as in outside nature, because it is found in the food and drink we take and then again in our elimination products—air, sweat, urine, faeces—and in secretions such as bile.

People do not feel the need today to ask what happens to the substance presenting as hydrogen before it enters into the organism and once it has been eliminated.

They do not ask: what does the substance presenting as hydrogen go through in the organism?

In raising the question one immediately feels the need to direct attention to the difference between the sleeping and the waking organism. The nature of a sleeping organism in terms of matter or substance does not provide a basis on which conscious and self-aware experiences can evolve. It does, however, provide a basis for life to evolve. In this respect a sleeping organism differs from a dead one. In the latter, the material basis no longer provides for life. We shall be unable to gain further understanding as long as we consider the difference to lie merely in a different composition of substances in a dead and a living organism.

Almost half a century ago the distinguished physiologist Emil Du Bois-Reymond[2] pointed out that conscious awareness will never be explained in terms of how substances act. He said people would never understand why it should not be a matter of indifference to a specific number of carbon, oxygen, nitrogen and hydrogen atoms how they are, were and will be positioned, and why with their change in position they cause a human being to feel: I see red; I smell the scent of roses. This being the case, Du Bois-Reymond said, people using the natural scientific approach would never be able to explain the waking human being who is full of feelings and sensations, but only the sleeping human being.

He was under an illusion in taking this view. He believed that the actions of substances gave rise to the phenomena not of consciousness but of life. In reality, however, we have to say the same for the phenomena of life as Du Bois-Reymond did for those of conscious awareness. Why should it occur to a number of carbon, oxygen, hydrogen and nitrogen atoms to produce the phenomena of life through the way they were, are or will be positioned?

Observation has shown that the phenomena of life have a completely different orientation from those that occur in the lifeless sphere. For the latter we may say: they show themselves to be governed by forces that radiate from the essential nature of the substance, from the—relative—centre to the periphery. The phenomena of life show matter to be governed by forces that act from outside in, towards the—relative—centre. In the transition to life, matter must withdraw from the outward radiating forces and make itself part of those that radiate in.

Every substance and also every process on earth has its forces that radiate out from the earth and holds them in common with the earth. It is the kind of substance chemists see merely as a constituent part of the earth's body. Entering into the sphere of life, it has to cease being merely part of the earth. It goes beyond having things in common with the earth. It is included in a sphere of forces that radiate towards the earth from the world beyond the earth that is all around. Seeing a substance or process evolve as life, we have to think of it as withdrawing from the forces that act on it as though from the centre of the earth and entering into the sphere of other forces that do not have a centre but a periphery.

They act from all directions, those forces, as though aiming for the centre of the earth. They would have to dissolve all that is matter on earth into utter formlessness, tearing it apart, if the influences of the heavenly bodies from beyond the earth's sphere did not enter into the space in which these forces are active and modify the dissolution. We can observe this if we study plants. In plants, earth substances are lifted out of the sphere of earth activities. They go in the direction of formlessness. This transition to formlessness is modified by the actions of the sun and similar effects from the cosmos. If these are not taking effect, or acting in a different way, e.g. during the night, the forces that substances have in common with the earth come alive in them again. Plant nature develops in the interaction of earthly and cosmic forces. If we call the whole sphere of forces that are under the earth's influence the 'physical', we shall need another name for the very different nature of the forces that do not radiate from the earth but radiate in towards it. Here an aspect of the human organization which we discussed in the previous chapter shows itself in a different light. In accord with an earlier usage that has been thrown into confusion under the influence of more recent physics-oriented thinking, we called this part of the human organism the etheric. We shall have to say that the etheric is active in plant nature, that is, in the sphere that presents as life.

In so far as the human being is a living entity, this etheric is also active in him. Yet even with regard to mere phenomena of life, there is a significant difference compared to plant nature. The plant allows the physical to be active in it when the etheric from cosmic space no longer takes effect, as is the case when the sun ether ceases to take effect during the night. Man only allows the physical to be active in his body in death. During sleep, the phenomena of conscious awareness and self awareness vanish; the phenomena of life continue, however, even when the sun ether is not actively at work in cosmic space. The plant is throughout its life taking in the ether forces radiating down on to the earth. Man has them inside himself in an individualized form even in his embryonic period. Thus man takes *out of himself* what the plant receives from the world, because he received it for his further development when still in his mother's womb. A power that is truly cosmic in origin, designed to act by radiating down on to the earth, is acting out of lung or liver. It has metamorphosed its direction.

We therefore have to say that human beings have the etheric in them and that it is individualized. The physical has been individualized in the form of the physical body and of its organs, and so has the etheric. Human beings have a distinct ether body and a distinct physical body. During sleep this ether body remains connected with the physical body, giving it life; it only separates from it in death.

4
On the Nature of the Sentient Organism

The form and organization of a plant results from two spheres of forces only: those that radiate from the earth and those that radiate towards it; the animal and human form and organizations do not result only from these. A plant leaf is exclusively under the influence of those two spheres of forces; the animal lung is also under their influence, but not exclusively so. For the leaf, all configuring forces lie *in* those spheres; for the lung, forces also exist that exist beyond these. This applies both to the configuring forces that create outer form and to those which regulate the inner movement of matter, giving it a specific direction and either combining or separating it.

We may say that for substances taken into the plant it is not a matter of indifference whether they live or do not live, for they enter into the sphere of forces radiating towards the earth. They are lifeless in the plant if the forces of the periphery do not act on them; they enter into life when they come under the influence of these forces.

Even alive, however, plant substance is indifferent to how its elements have been, are or will be positioned with reference to their own activity. They give themselves up to the activity of outward and inward radiating external forces. Animal substance comes under influences that are independent of these forces. It moves within the organism, or as a whole organism, in such a way that these movements do not follow from the outward and inward radiating forces only. Because of this, animal configuration is independent of the spheres of forces radiating from or towards the earth.

In the plant, the interplay of those forces results in alternation between being subject to the forces radiating in from the periphery and not being subject to them. This divides plant nature into two aspects. One is oriented towards life, it is wholly in the sphere of the periphery; these are the sprouting organs that sustain growth and flower. The other is oriented toward the lifeless, it remains in the sphere of outward radiating forces, it includes everything that hardens growth, providing a firm supporting structure for life, etc. Between these two aspects life ignites and dies away; and the dying of a plant is merely the dominance of outward radiating over inward radiating forces.

In the animal, part of the substantial element is completely withdrawn from the influence of the two spheres of forces. The resulting differentiation differs from that of plants. Organs develop that remain within the influence of both spheres of forces, and also organs that lie outside them. Interactions arise between the two types of organ development. And it is due to *these* interactions that animal substance can be the vehicle for feeling and sensation. One consequence is the difference in the appearance, the consistency of animal compared to plant substance.

In the animal organism we have one sphere of forces that is independent of those radiating from the earth and radiating towards it. The astral sphere of forces is present in addition to the physical and etheric; we have already referred to this from another point of view. No need to be put off by the term 'astral'. The outward radiating forces are those of the earth, the inward radiating forces those of the earth's cosmic periphery; in the 'astral' forces lies something of a higher order than those two. It is this alone which makes the earth a cosmic body, a 'star' (*astrum*). Through the physical forces it separates itself from the cosmos, through the etheric forces it lets the cosmos influence it; through the 'astral' forces it becomes an independent individual entity in the cosmos.

Like the etheric and the physical body, the 'astral' in the animal organism is an independent, self-contained aspect. We may therefore speak of this aspect as the 'astral body'.

We can only understand the animal organization if we consider the interrelationships between physical, etheric and astral body. All three are independent aspects of the animal organization; and all three are also different from what exists in the lifeless (mineral) bodies and the living plant organisms outside them.

The animal physical organism may be said to be life-less; it differs, however, from lifeless mineral elements. It is first estranged from the mineral sphere by the etheric and astral organism, and then, through withdrawal of the etheric and astral forces, given back to the lifeless sphere. It is a structure in which the forces that are active in the mineral sphere, in the earth realm as such, can only be destructive. It can only serve the animal organism as a whole for as long as the etheric and astral forces prevail over the destructive intervention of the mineral sphere.

The animal etheric organism lives like the plant organism, but not in the same way. Life is taken to a state that is foreign to itself by the astral forces; it has been torn away from the forces radiating inward to the earth and then placed in their sphere again. The etheric organism is a structure in which merely plant-type forces are at a level of existence that is too dull or dim for the animal organization. It can only serve the animal organism as a whole in so far as the astral forces raise its mode of action to a brighter level; if it gains the upper hand in its activities, sleep ensues; if the astral organism gains the upper hand, waking prevails.

Both sleeping and waking must not go beyond certain levels of activity. If this were to happen in the case of sleep, the plant principle in the organism as a whole would tend towards the mineral; the plant principle would hypertrophy, which would be a pathological condition. If it happened in the case of waking, the plant principle would have to become completely estranged from the mineral; this would assume forms in the organism that are not its own but belong to the lifeless sphere which lies outside the organic. A pathological condition would develop due to hypertrophy of the mineral principle.

Physical substance enters from outside into all three organisms—physical, etheric and astral. All three must overcome the inherent nature of the physical in their own way. This results in a threefold differentiation of organs. The physical organization creates organs that have gone through the etheric and astral organization but are on the way back to its sphere. They cannot have arrived in its sphere completely; for that would result in death of the organism.

The etheric organism creates organs that have gone through the astral organization but continually seek to withdraw from it; they have the power to enter into the dimness of sleep; they tend to evolve purely vegetative life.

The astral organism creates organs that alienate themselves from vegetative life. They can only continue to exist if this vegetative life is continually taking hold of them again. Having no relationship with the forces that radiate from and towards the earth, they would have to drop out completely from the earthly sphere if this did not continually take hold of them again. There has to be rhythmic interaction between animal and plant principles in these organs. This determines the alternating states of sleeping and waking. In sleep, the organs of the astral forces are also in the dimness of vegetable life. There they have no influence on the etheric and physical spheres. These are then entirely left to the spheres of forces that radiate from and towards the earth.

5
Plant, Animal, Man

In the astral body, animal configuration arises as a whole form on the outside and inwardly as the configuration of the organs. And sentient animal substance is one result of this configuring astral body. If this configuration is taken to its conclusion, the animal principle is created.

In man it is not taken to its conclusion. It is brought to a halt, inhibited, at a certain point along the road.

In the plant, we have substance which is transformed by the forces that radiate inwards on to the earth. This is living substance. It is in interaction with lifeless substance. We have to see that in plant nature this living substance is continually separated out from lifeless substance. In it, the plant form appears as the outcome of the forces that radiate towards the earth. This results in a stream of substance. Lifeless principles are transformed into live; live principles become lifeless. Within this stream plant organs arise.

In the animal sentient substance arises from live substance, just as in the plant live substance arises from the lifeless. A twofold substance stream exists. Life is not taken to fully configured life within the etheric. It remains in a state of flux; and the configuring process enters into this flowing life through the astral organization.

In man, *this* process, too, is kept in a state of flux. Sentient substance is drawn into the sphere of yet another organization. We may call this the I organization. Sentient substance changes once again. A threefold substance stream results. In this arises the inner and outer human form. This makes it the vehicle of a self-aware life in mind and spirit. In his configuration man is the outcome of this I organization down to the smallest particles of his substance.

It is possible to study the substance aspect of this configuration. When substance is transformed from one level to the next, it presents as the higher level separated off from the lower, with the configuration created from the substance that has been separated off. In the plant, living substance is separated off from lifeless substance. In this secreted substance the etheric forces that radiate in towards the Earth are at work as configuring forces. Initially there is no actual separating off but complete transformation of the physical substance by the etheric forces. This, however, is only the case in seed development. Here the transformation can be complete because the seed is protected from the influences of physical forces by the enveloping maternal organization. When seed development frees itself from the maternal organization, the activity of forces in the plant is differentiated into one where substance creation goes in the direction of the etheric sphere and one where it goes in the direction of physical development. Parts of plant nature develop which are on the path of life, and others that go in the direction of death. These present as excreted parts of the plant organism. The excretion process can be seen in bark production in trees, which is a highly characteristic example.

In the animal, twofold separation is in progress and also twofold excretion. Plant secretion is not taken to its conclusion but kept in a state of flux, and added to this is the transformation of living into sentient substance. This separates off from merely living substance. We have substance that goes in the direction of sentient nature and substance that goes away from this and in the direction of mere life.

There is, however, interaction of all parts in the organism. Because of this, excretion in the direction of the lifeless sphere, which in the plant approaches to the external, mineral lifeless sphere, is still far removed from this mineral sphere. In bark production, substance is created in plants that is on the way to being mineral and separates off the more mineral it becomes. In the animal world, this principle appears as the excretion products of digestion. It is further removed from the mineral sphere than the plant secretion.

In man, the substance separated off from sentient substance becomes the vehicle for the self-aware mind and spirit. But there is also continuous secretion, with a substance produced that goes in the direction of pure capacity for sentience. The animal principle exists as continuous excretion within the human organism.

In the waking state of the animal organism, separating off and configuration of material that has been separated off as well as secretion of sentient substance are under the influence of astral activity. In man, the activity of the I organism is added to this. During sleep, astral and I organism take no direct action. But the substance has been taken hold of by this activity and continues it as though seeking to maintain inertia. Once a substance has been inwardly configured the way it is by astral and I organization, it will continue to act in terms of these organizations in the sleeping state, reflecting a capacity for inertia.

In a human being who is asleep we thus cannot speak of purely vegetative function in the organism. The astral and the I organization continue to be active in the substance they have configured even in this state. The difference between sleeping and waking is not one of alternation between human-animalic and vegetative-physical function. The situation is entirely different. Sentient substance and substance capable of supporting the self-aware mind and spirit are lifted out of the total organism on waking and put at the service of the astral body and I organization. The physical and the etheric organism must then function in such a way that only the forces radiating out from the earth and radiating in towards it are active in them. In this mode of action they are only taken hold of from the outside by the astral body and I organization. During sleep, however, they are inwardly taken hold of by the substances that develop under the influence of the astral body and the I organization. While only the forces radiating out from the earth and radiating in towards it act from the universe on a sleeping person, the substance-forces created by the astral body and the I organization are working on that person from within.

If we call sentient substance the *residue* of the astral body and the substance developed under the influence of the I organization the *residue* of *that* organization, we are able to say: in the waking human organism, the astral body and the I organization themselves are active, in the sleeping organism their substantial residues are active.

Waking, human beings live in an activity that connects them with the outside world through their astral body and their I organization; sleeping, their physical and their etheric organism live on what the residues of these two organizations have become in terms of substance. The actions of a substance like oxygen, which is taken in through respiration both in the sleeping and in the waking state, therefore have to be seen as having different effects in these two states. The nature of oxygen taken in from outside is such that it has a hypnotic, not a stimulating effect. Increased oxygen intake makes us abnormally sleepy. In the waking state the astral body is continually fighting the hypnotic action of oxygen intake. If the astral body ceases to act on the physical body, oxygen develops its inherent quality: it makes us go to sleep.

6
Blood and Nerve

The functions of individual human organisms with reference to the total organism are particularly well demonstrated in blood and nerve development. Blood production consists in further configuration of the foods that have been taken in, with the whole process under the influence of the I organization. The I organization influences functions ranging from those that accompany conscious sensation—in the tongue, in the palate—to those occurring at an unconscious or subconscious level—the actions of pepsin, pancreas, bile, etc. The activity of the I organization then lessens, and the astral body is predominantly active in further transforming food substance into blood substance. This continues until the blood encounters the air—the oxygen—in the respiratory process. This is where the ether body plays its main role. Carbon dioxide that is in the process of exhalation is essentially live substance—not sentient and not dead—before it leaves the body. (Everything that has ether body activity in it is live.) The main part of this live carbon dioxide leaves the organism; a small part continues to be active in the organism, influencing processes that have their focus in the head organization. This part shows a marked tendency to become lifeless, inorganic, though it does not become completely lifeless.

The opposite is the case in the nervous system. The etheric body is predominantly active in the sympathetic nervous system, which is present throughout the digestive organs. The nerve organs concerned are essentially organs that are live by nature. The astral and the I organization do not organize them from inside but from outside. This means that the influence of the I and astral organization active in these nerve organs is powerful. Affects and passions have a continuous, significant effect on the sympathetic system. Worry and cares will gradually destroy it.

The astral organization is predominantly active in the nervous system in the spinal marrow with all its branches. This makes it the vehicle for the soul aspect of the human being, of reflex processes, but not for anything that happens in the I, in the self-aware mind and spirit.

The actual cerebral nerves are the ones that are subject to the I organization. In them the activities of the etheric and astral organization are less marked.

We see that this results in three regions within the sphere of the total organism. We have a lower region where the nerves, which are inwardly predominantly organized by the etheric organism, act together with the blood substance, which is essentially subject to the activity of the I organization. In the embryonic and post-embryonic stages of development this region is where the development begins of all organs connected with inner quickening of the human organism. As the embryo develops, this region, which is still weak at the time, is supplied with quickening and creative influences from the maternal organism that surrounds it. Then there is a middle region where nerve organs influenced by the astral organization act together with blood processes, which are also dependent on this astral organization and in their upper part on the etheric organization. During the human development period this is where the genesis of organs begins that mediate external and internal mobility, e.g. for all muscle development and also all organs that whilst not actual muscles nevertheless bring about mobility.—An upper region exists where the nerves subject to inner organization by the I act together with the blood processes that have a powerful tendency to become lifeless, mineral. During the human development period this is where the development of bone and everything else begins that serves the human body by way of structural supportive organs.

We shall only be able to understand the human brain if we see in it a bone-developing tendency that is interrupted in its earliest incipient stage. And we shall only be able to understand bone development if we perceive in it a brain-impulse activity that has completely come to an end and is penetrated from outside by the impulses of the middle organism where astrally determined nerve organs are active together with etherically determined blood substance. In bone ash, which retains its own inherent configuration when bones are put through a combustion process, we have the products of the uppermost region in the human organization. In the cartilaginous substance which remains when bones are treated with dilute hydrochloric acid we have the product of the impulses from the middle region.

The skeleton is the physical image of the I organization. Human organic substance that seeks to become lifeless and mineral is completely subject to the I organization in bone development. In the brain, the I is active as a spiritual entity. There, however, its form-generating power, which influences the physical, is completely overcome by etheric organizing processes, and indeed by the inherent forces of the physical. The organizing power of the I is minimal in the brain; it is swamped by life processes and by physical processes following their inherent laws. This is the true reason why the brain is the vehicle for mental and spiritual I activity, that in it, organic, physical activity is not subject to the I organization, which is therefore able to act in complete freedom. The bony skeleton on the other hand is the complete physical image of the I organization; this, however, exhausts itself in its physical organizing activities, so that nothing remains of it by way of mental or spiritual activity. The processes in our bones are therefore the most unconscious.

The carbon dioxide which is pushed out in the respiratory process is still live substance when within the organism; it is taken hold of by the astral activity which is anchored in the middle nervous system and eliminated to the outside. The part of the carbon dioxide that goes with the metabolism to the head is there combined with calcium and thus given the inclination to enter into the activities of the I organization. In this way, calcium carbonate is pushed in the direction of bone development under the influence of head nerves given their inner impulses by the I organization.

Two substances produced from our food—myosin and myogen—have a tendency to become deposited in the blood; they are initially astrally determined and in interaction with the sympathetic nervous system, which is inwardly organized by the etheric body. These two proteins are, however, also partly taken hold of by the activity of the middle nervous system, which is under the influence of the astral body. Because of this they enter into relationship with protein decomposition products, with fats, with sugars and sugar-like substances. This enables them to go in the direction of muscle development under the influence of the middle nervous system.

7
The Nature of Medicinal Actions

The total human organization is not a self-contained system of interactive processes. If it were, it could not be the vehicle for the element of soul and spirit. This can only have the human organism as its base because the organism is continually decomposing or going in the direction of lifeless, mineral activity in its nerve and bone substance and in the processes of which those substances are a part.

Protein substance decomposes in nerve tissue. It is not recreated, however, by entering into the sphere of the forces that radiate in towards the earth, as in the ovum or other structures, but simply decomposes. As a result ether activities radiating in from objects and events in the outer environment through the senses, and ether activities created when the organs of movement are used, are able to utilize the nerves as organs along which they are conducted through the whole body.

There are two kinds of processes in nerves: the decomposition of proteins and the flow of ether substance through the decomposing substance, a flow fanned to life by acids, salts, phosphorous and sulphurous principles. The balance between the two processes is mediated by fats and water.

By nature these processes are pathological processes continually present throughout the organism. They have to be balanced out by equally continuous healing processes.

Balance is achieved because the blood contains not only processes of growth and metabolism but also a continual *healing* activity that counterbalances the pathological processes in the nerves.

In the plasma substance and fibrous material of the blood lie the forces that serve growth and metabolism in the narrower sense. In the iron content which is found when we examine red blood cells lie the origins of the blood's *healing* activity. Because of this, iron is also found in gastric juice and as iron oxide in chyle. There sources are created everywhere for processes that have a balancing effect on the processes in the nerves.

If we examine the blood, iron is found to be the only metal which has the tendency to be crystallizable within the human organism. The forces it thus brings to bear are external, physical and mineral forces of nature. Within the human organism these represent a system of forces oriented in terms of outer physical nature. This, however, is continually overcome by the I organization.

We are dealing with two systems of forces. One has its origin in the processes that occur in nerves; the other in blood production. The processes in the nerves give rise to pathological processes which go so far that they can be continually healed by the blood processes that act in the opposite direction. The processes in the nerves are such as are brought about by the astral body in nerve substance and hence in the whole organism. The blood processes are such that in them the I organization inside the human organism confronts physical outside nature, which continues on into the organism but is forced into the configuration imposed by the I organization.

This interrelationship provides direct insight into the processes of disease and healing. If processes the normal level of which is determined by what is excited by the nerve-type process are enhanced, it is a case of disease. If we are able to oppose these processes with others that represent an enhancement of external natural activities in the organism, healing can be achieved if these external natural activities are under the control of the I organism and serve to balance out the processes that have the opposite orientation.

Milk contains only small amounts of iron. It is the substance which as such is the least likely to cause pathological changes; the blood must constantly submit to everything potentially pathological; it therefore needs iron that has been organized, i.e. made part of the I organization—haem—as a continual medicine.

When a medicine is to influence a pathological condition developing in the inner organization, even if this is due to external causes though it develops in the inner organism, it is first of all important to see in how far the astral organization is acting to the effect that protein decomposition occurs somewhere in the organism in such a way that it is initiated in the normal way by the nerve organization. Let us assume we are dealing with stasis in the lower abdomen. The pain which develops may be noted to be excessive activity of the astral body. We are thus dealing with the characterized situation in the intestinal organism.

The next important question is: how can the increased astral activity be balanced out? This may be done by introducing substances into the blood that may be taken hold of by the part of the I organization that is active in the intestinal organization. These are potassium and sodium. If these are introduced into the organism in the form of a preparation, or in a plant organization such as

Anagallis arvensis, the astral body is relieved of its excessive nerve activity, with the excess astral activity transferred to the activity of the above-mentioned substances which have been taken hold of from the I, an activity that arises out of the blood.

If we use the mineral substance, care will have to be taken to add other substances or, even better, combine the potassium or sodium with sulphur in the preparation, so that these metals are introduced into the bloodstream in a way that stops protein metamorphosis before decomposition sets in. Sulphur has the property of serving to stop protein decomposition; it may be said to hold the organizing forces together in the protein substance. If it enters into the bloodstream in potassium or sodium compounds its action will be directed to areas where potassium or sodium are specially attracted to specific organs. This is the case with the intestinal organs.

8

Activities in the Human Organism

Diabetes mellitus

The human organism evolves activities through all its constituent parts that can only have their impulses within the organism as such. Anything taken in from outside must either merely be something that enables it to develop its own activity; or it has to act in such a way in the body that the foreign activity does not differ from one of the body's own inner activities once it has entered into the body.

The food human beings need contains carbohydrates, for instance. These are partly starchlike. As such they are substances that develop their activity in the plant. They enter into the human body in the state they are able to achieve in the plant. In this state, starch is a foreign body. The human organism does not evolve any activity that goes in the direction of what starch is able to evolve as an activity when it enters into the body. Thus the starchlike material developed in the human liver (glycogen) is different from vegetable starch. Glucose on the other hand is a substance that stimulates activities which are of the same kind as activities of the human organism. Starch therefore must not continue as starch in the human organism. If it is to evolve an activity that plays a role in the body, it must first be transformed. Mixed with ptyalin in the oral cavity it is converted to sugar.

Protein and fat are not changed by ptyalin. They are

initially foreign matter as they enter the stomach. Here the protein is transformed by the pepsin secreted in the stomach, producing cleavage products that go as far as the peptones. These are substances the activity impulses of which coincide with those of the body. Fat, however, remains unchanged even in the stomach. It is finally transformed by the product separated off by the pancreas and substances are obtained that result from the dead organism as glycerine and fatty acids.

The conversion of starch into sugars occurs throughout the digestive process. Starch that has not been converted by ptyalin will also be converted by the gastric juice.

If starch is converted by ptyalin, the process is on the borderline for anything that occurs in the sphere of the I organization, as we called it in chapter 2. The first conversion of what has been taken in from outside takes place in its sphere. Glucose is a substance able to be active in the sphere of the I organization. It relates to the taste of sweetness, which has its being in the I organization.

If starch flour is converted to sugar by the gastric juice, this signifies that the I organization penetrates into the sphere of the digestive system. The taste of sweetness does not become conscious in that case; instead the process, which happens in the conscious mind—in the sphere of the I organization—when 'sweet' is experienced, enters into the unconscious regions of the human body and the I organization becomes active there.

In the terms established in chapter 2, it is first of all the astral body which is active in the unconscious regions. It is active where starch is converted to sugars in the stomach.

We can only have conscious awareness through a process in our I organization which is such that the organization is not drowned out or disturbed by anything else and is able to come fully into its own. This is the case in the sphere where ptyalin activities occur. In the sphere of pepsin activities the astral body drowns out the I organization. I activity becomes immersed in astral activity. It is thus possible to trace the I organization in the material sphere by the presence of sugar. Where you have sugar, you have I organization; where sugar is produced, the I organization comes on the scene and gives subhuman (vegetative, animalic) bodily nature an orientation towards humanity.

Sugar occurs as an elimination product in diabetes mellitus. This is a case of the I organization coming on the scene in the human organism in such a form that its actions are destructive. If we consider any other region of I organization activity we find that it becomes immersed in the astral organization. Consumed as it is, sugar is in the I organization. It causes the sweet taste to develop. Starch which is ingested and converted to sugar by ptyalin or the gastric juice indicates that the astral body is working together with the I organization in the oral cavity or stomach and drowning it out.

Sugar is also found in the blood. Because the blood contains sugar as it circulates throughout the whole body it carries the I organization to all parts of it. Yet wherever it goes this I organization is kept in balance by the activity of the human organism. We have seen in chapter 2 that in addition to the I organization and the astral body the essential human being also contains the etheric and the physical body. These, too, take the I organization into themselves and hold it there. For as long as this is the case, the urine does not separate off sugar. The sugar-related processes in the organism show us how the I organization, as the vehicle for sugar, is able to live.

In a healthy individual sugar will only appear in the urine if too much has been taken, or if too much alcohol has been taken, for this enters directly into our bodily processes, not going through intermediary product stages first. In either case the sugar process is independent of other processes in the human being.

With diabetes mellitus the situation is that the I organization is weakened to such a degree as it enters into the astral and etheric sphere that it is no longer able to apply its activity to the sugar substance. What should have happened to the sugar through the I organization then happens to it through the astral and etheric regions.

Anything which tears the I organization away from its activities that intervene in bodily functions will encourage diabetes: upsets that are not single but repeated events; intellectual overexertion; a hereditary trait that prevents normal incorporation of the I organization in the total organism. All this is also connected with the fact that processes take place in the head organization that should really run parallel to activity in soul and spirit; but because this activity is too fast or to slow the processes cease to be parallel. The nervous system is, as it were, thinking independently alongside the thinking human being. This, however, is an activity the nervous system should perform only in sleep. In diabetics, a kind of sleep deep down in the organism runs parallel to the waking state. As a result, degeneration of nerve substance occurs with diabetes. It is the consequence of inadequate intervention from the I organization.

Another symptom diabetics have is that they develop

boils. Boils develop through excess in the region of etheric activity. The I organization fails to act where it should. Astral activity cannot evolve because in such a site in particular it can only take effect in harmony with the I organization. The consequence is the excess of etheric activity that comes to expression in boils.

It is evident from all this that a healing process can only be initiated in diabetes if we are able to strengthen the I organization of the diabetic.

9
The Role of Protein in the Human Body and Proteinuria

Protein is the substance in the living body that can be transformed in the greatest variety of ways by its creative etheric forces, so that the forms of organs and of the organism as a whole are the outcome of protein trans-formation. To be used in such a way, protein must have the ability to lose any form resulting from the nature of its material parts the moment it is called upon to serve a form that is demanded of it in the organism.

It is evident from this that the forces deriving from the nature of the hydrogen, oxygen, nitrogen and carbon and their interrelations collapse within protein. Inorganic bonds cease to exist, and forces creating organic forms begin to be active in protein decomposition.

These creative forces are bound to the etheric body. Protein is always on the point of either being taken up into the activity of the etheric body or of dropping out of it. Protein taken out of the organism to which it belonged assumes the tendency to become a composite subject to the inorganic forces of hydrogen, oxygen, nitrogen and carbon. Protein that remains part of the living organism suppresses this tendency and submits to the creative powers of the etheric body.

We take in protein with our food. Gastric pepsin converts protein taken in from outside into peptones, initially soluble proteins. Conversion then continues with the aid of pancreatic juice.

Initially the protein taken in as food is a foreign body in the human organism. It contains the after-effects of the ether processes of the life form from which it has been taken. These must be completely removed. The protein has to be taken into the ether activities of the human organism.

We thus have two kinds of protein within the human digestive process. At the beginning of the process the protein is something foreign to the human organism. At the end it is something the organism has made its own. In between lies a state where the food protein has not yet entirely let go of those earlier ether activities and has not yet entirely taken in the new ones. It has become almost inorganic in this state. It is the point where it is solely under the influence of the human physical body. This, which in its form is a product of the human I organization, has in it the powers to act inorganically. It thus acts to kill anything that lives. Everything that comes within the sphere of the I organization dies off. The I organization thus incorporates purely inorganic substances into itself in the physical body. These do not act in the human physical organism the way they do in lifeless nature outside the human being; but their action is inorganic, i.e. they kill. This death-inducing action is applied to protein at the point in the digestive region where trypsin is active, a constituent of pancreatic juice.—

The trypsin mode of action also involves inorganic principles, as can be seen from the fact that this substance develops its activity with the aid of alkaline principles.

Food protein lives in a foreign manner until it encounters the trypsin of the pancreas; it lives in the mode of the organism from which it has been taken. On encountering trypsin, the protein becomes lifeless. One might say that it only becomes lifeless for a moment in the human organism. There it is taken up into the physical body in accord with the principles of the I organization. This must have the power to transfer the converted protein into the sphere of the human ether body. Food protein thus becomes material for the creation of the human organism. The foreign etheric activities formerly attached to it leave the human being.

To digest protein in a healthy way, human beings need an I organization which is so strong that all the protein needed for the human organism can be transferred to the sphere of the human ether body. If this is not the case, this ether body develops excessive activity. It does not receive enough protein prepared by the I organization for its activity. The consequence is that the activity oriented towards enlivening protein taken in by the I organization takes hold of protein that still contains foreign ether activities. The human being receives a number of activities in the ether body that do not belong there. These have to be eliminated in an irregular way. The result is pathological elimination.

This pathological elimination takes the form of *proteinuria*. Protein is eliminated that should be taken up into the sphere of the ether body. It is protein which because of weakness in the I organization has not been able to assume the transitional state of being almost lifeless.

The forces that effect elimination in the human being are bound to the sphere of the astral body. With proteinuria the astral body is forced to perform a function for which it is not prepared, and this causes its function to diminish in the areas where it should develop in the human organism. This is in the renal epithelium.

Damage to the renal epithelium is a symptom indicating that the astral activity designed for it has been deflected.

It is evident from the above where healing has to begin in the case of proteinuria. The power of the I organization needs to be strengthened in the pancreas where it is too weak.

10
The Role of Fat in the Human Organism and Deceptive Local Symptom Complexes

Fat proves least of a foreign substance when taken into the organism. Fat will most easily change from the nature it has when taken in as food to the nature of the human organism. The 80 per cent of fat contained in butter, for instance, goes unchanged through the ptyalin and pepsin regions and is only changed by pancreatic juice, converting to glycerine and fatty acids.

Fat is able to behave like this because it takes as little as possible of a foreign organism's nature (its etheric forces, etc.) into the human organism. The human organism can easily make it part of its own sphere of activity.

The reason is that fat plays a special role in producing inner warmth. This warmth is the element in which the I organization predominantly lives, i.e. as a physical organism. With *every* substance in the human body, relevance to the I organization is limited to as much of it as develops heat in its activity. In the whole way it behaves, fat proves to be a substance that merely fills the body, being merely carried by it, being of relevance to the active organization only because of the processes in which heat evolves. Fat taken for food from an animal organism, for instance, will take nothing but its ability to evolve heat into the human organism.

The evolution of heat is, however, one of the processes that come last in metabolism. Fat taken in as food therefore stays as it is in the early and the middle metabolic processes, and is only taken up into the sphere of inner bodily activity at the earliest by pancreatic juice.

The presence of fat in human milk points to a highly remarkable activity in the organism. The body does not inwardly consume this fat; it lets it become a product that is separated off. This means, however, that the I organization also becomes part of *this* fat. The power to be open to creative impulses that is found in mother's milk depends on this. The mother transfers her own I organization's powers of being open to creative impulses to the child, thus adding something further to the powers of configuration transmitted by heredity.

A healthy route is given if the human form-generating powers consume the fat available in the body in the process of generating heat. An unhealthy route is given if the fat is not used up in heat generation by the I organization but taken unused into the organism. Such fat creates excess potential for the generation of heat in one place or another in the organism. This heat intervenes here and there in the organism and causes confusion for the other vital processes, not being encompassed by the I organization. Parasitic heat foci develop, as it were. These have a tendency to produce inflammatory conditions. The genesis of such foci must be seen to be due to the body developing the tendency to produce more fat than the I organization needs for its life in inner warmth.

In a healthy organism, animalic (astral) forces produce or take in as much fat as can be converted to heat processes by the I organization, and in addition the amount needed to keep muscle and bone mechanics in good order. In this case, the warmth needed for the body will be produced. If the animalic forces provide too little fat for the I organization, the I organization develops a hunger for warmth. It has to draw the warmth it needs from the activities of organs. This causes them to become friable and stiff in themselves, as it were. The processes they need become sluggish. One then sees pathological processes developing here and there, and we have to discern if they are due to a general fat deficiency.

If the opposite is the case, and there is excess fat content, as already mentioned, so that parasitic heat foci develop, organs are taken hold of in such a way that they become excessively active. This creates tendencies to excessive food intake, overloading the body. It is not at all necessary for this development to take the form of the individual concerned becoming an over-eater. It may be, for instance, that too much substance it taken to a head organ as part of metabolic activity in the organism, being therefore withdrawn from the abdominal organs and separating off processes. As a result, the activity of those badly supplied organs is reduced. Material separated off by the glands may be deficient. The fluid constituents of the organism fall into unhealthy relative proportions. Thus separated-off bile may be excessive relative to material separated off by the pancreas. Again it will be a question of discerning how a local symptom complex should be judged concerning its origin in unhealthy fat activity.

11
The Configuration of the Human Body and Gout

Protein uptake is a process connected with *one* aspect of the inner activities in the human organism. It is the aspect that arises on the basis of assimilation of matter. Any activity of this kind results in the development of form, in growth, new development of substantial content. Everything connected with the unconscious functions of the organism belongs to this.

These processes are in contrast to processes involving elimination. Eliminations may go outside the body; but there are also processes where the elimination product is processed further inside in giving the body form or substance. These processes are the material basis for conscious experiences. Processes of the first kind reduce the power of consciousness if they go beyond the level that can be held in balance by the processes of the second kind.

A particularly remarkable elimination process is that of uric acid. The astral body is active in this elimination. The process has to happen throughout the whole organism. It happens to a particular degree via the urine. In a subtly dispersed form in the brain, for instance. The astral body is mainly involved when uric acid is eliminated via the urine; the I organization plays a lesser role. When uric acid is separated off in the brain, the I organization is the main determiner, the astral body taking a less active role.

In the organism, the astral body mediates I organization activity for the etheric and physical body. The I
organization has to transport the lifeless substances and
forces to the organs. It is only by thus impregnating the
organs with inorganic principles that human beings can
be the conscious life form they are. Organic substance
and organic energy would reduce human consciousness
to the animal level.

The astral body is active in a way that makes the
organs inclined to accept the inorganic deposits of the I
organization. It prepares the way for this, as it were.

We see that astral body activity has the upper hand in
the lower parts of the human organism. There, the uric
acid substances must not be taken up by the organism.
They must be abundantly eliminated. There, impregnation with inorganic principles must be prevented under
the influence of this elimination process. The more uric
acid is eliminated the more lively is the function of the
astral body, the less is I organization activity and hence
impregnation with inorganic principles.

In the brain, astral body activity is minimal. Little uric
acid is eliminated, but all the more inorganic principles
are deposited in accord with the nature of the I organization.

The I organization cannot deal with large amounts of
uric acid; they must be left to the activity of the astral
body; small amounts of uric acid become part of the I
organization to provide the basis for shaping the inorganic in accord with the nature of this organization.

Uric acid distribution in the different regions of the
healthy organism has to be managed in exactly the right
way. The amount of uric acid provided for everything
connected with the organization of nerves and senses

should be no more than can be used in I activity; this activity has to be suppressed for the organization of metabolism and limbs; astral activity must be able to develop in abundant uric acid elimination.

Since the astral body prepares the way for I activity in the organs, the proper distribution of uric acid deposits must be considered to be a highly important aspect of human health. It is an expression indicating if the right relationship exists between I organization and astral body in any organ or organ system.

Let us assume astral activity is gaining the upper hand in an organ where the I organization should predominate over it. This can only be an organ designed in such a way that uric acid elimination cannot go beyond a certain limit. Now the organ is overloaded with uric acid that has not been dealt with by the I organization. The astral body then starts to bring about elimination after all. And as efferent organs are not available at the relevant points, the uric acid does not go outside but is deposited in the organism itself. If it reaches sites in the organism where the I organization is not able to intervene sufficiently, something inorganic will be there, i.e. principles that belong to the I organization only but are left to astral activity by that organization. Foci arise where subhuman (animal) processes are introduced into the human organism.

That is the situation we have with *gout*. When people say it frequently develops on the basis of heredity, this is because the astral, animal principle becomes particularly active if hereditary forces are dominant, and the I organization is pushed into the background.

We shall get a clearer picture, however, if we look for the true cause in the fact that substances are taken into the human organism with the food which cannot lose their foreign nature within the organism, through its activities. They are not transferred to the ether body if the I organization is weak, and remain in the region of astral activity. An articular cartilage or connective tissue structure can only be overloaded with uric acid, which causes an excess of inorganic principles in them, if I activity lags behind astral activity in those parts of the body. As the whole form of the human organism is a product of the I organization, the irregularity which has been described must cause deformation of the organs. The human organism seeks to abandon its form.

12
Development and Separating-off Processes of the Human Organism

Like other organisms, the human body develops from a semi-fluid state. Development always requires a supply of gaseous substances, however. The most important of these is oxygen, which is provided via the breathing process.

Let us first of all consider a solid part, e.g. a bone structure. It is secreted from the semi-fluid element. The I organization is active in this process of secretion. Anyone can see this if they follow the development of the skeletal system. It evolves to the degree to which the individual gains his human form as an expression of the I organization in the embryonic and childhood periods. The conversion of protein, which is the basis of this, initially involves removal of the (astral and etheric) foreign forces from the protein. The protein goes through an inorganic state; it has to become fluid in the process. In this state it is taken hold of by the I organization, which is active in warmth, and made part of the specifically human ether body. It becomes human protein. There is a long way to go yet before it becomes bone substance.

Following conversion into human protein it has to mature so that it can take in and give new form to calcium carbonate, phosphate, etc. This requires an intermediary stage. It has to come under the influence of the process in which gaseous matter is taken in. This brings the carbohydrate transformation products into the protein. Substances result that can provide the basis for the development of individual organs. These are not ready-made organ-specific substances such as liver or bone substance, but a more general substance from which all the individual organs of the body can be developed. The I organization is active in creating the final configuration of organs. The astral body is active in the above-mentioned, as yet undifferentiated organ substance. In the animal, this astral body also takes it upon itself to create the final configuration of organs; in man, astral body activity and hence animal nature only provides the general background for the I organization. Animal development is not taken to its conclusion in man; its progress is interrupted, with the human aspect imposed on it, as it were, by the I organization.

This I organization lives entirely in states of warmth. It evolves the individual organs out of the general astrality. The way it works on the general substance provided by the astral principle is to either increase or decrease the state of warmth in an organ preparing to come into existence.

If it reduces it, inorganic substances are in a hardening process as they enter into the substance and the basis for bone development is given. Salt substances are taken up.

If it increases it, organs are developed the function of which is to dissolve the organic, taking it into the fluid or gaseous state.

Let us assume the I organization finds that the organism has not developed the amount of warmth that would allow the state of warmth to be adequately increased for the organs that need this. The result is that organs whose activity should go in the direction of dis-solution develop hardening activity. A tendency that is healthy in bones becomes a pathological tendency in them.

Bone, when it has been formed out by the I organization, is an organ that is released from its sphere by the I organization. It enters into a state where it is no longer inwardly taken hold of by the I organization but only in an external way. It is taken out of the sphere of growth and organization and now merely serves the I organization in a mechanical capacity, performing the movements of the body. Only a residue of inner I organization activity persists in it throughout life, for it has to remain part of the organization within the organism and must not drop out of life.

The organs that for the above-mentioned reason may enter into bone-like development are the arteries. This results in calcification (sclerosis). The I organization is driven out of these organ systems, as it were.

The opposite is the case when the I organization does not find the reduction in the warmth state that is necessary for the skeletal sphere. The bones then become similar to the organs that develop dissolving activity. Due to lack of hardening they cannot provide a basis for the incorporation of salts. The final evolution of bony structures, which lies in the sphere of the I organization, thus fails to take place. Astral activity is not stopped at the right point along the way. Tendencies to malformation must result; for healthy configuration can only develop in the sphere of the I organization.

These are the conditions known as rickets. It can be seen from all this how human organs relate to their functions. Bone develops in the sphere of the I organization. When development has reached its conclusion, it serves this I organization which from now on no longer develops it but uses it to effect voluntary movements. The same applies to anything that evolves in the sphere of the astral organization. Here undifferentiated substances and forces are created. These occur throughout the body as the basis for differentiated organ development. Astral activity takes them to a certain level; after that it uses them. The whole human organism is permeated with semi-fluid material in which astrally oriented activity takes place.

This activity lives in separating off materials which are utilized to develop the organism in the direction of its higher aspects. Matter separated off in that direction has to be recognized in glandular products that play a role in the economy of the organism and its functions. Apart from these separated-off materials, which go inward in the organism, there are others which are actual eliminations to the outside. It would be wrong to see no more in them than parts of the food taken in for which the organism has no use, therefore ejecting it. What matters is not that the organism separates material off to the outside, but that it performs the functions which result in elimination. The performance of these functions holds an element which the organism *needs* to maintain itself. *This* activity is just as necessary as the one which consists in taking matter into the organism or depositing it within it. The essential nature of organic function lies in a healthy relationship between these *two* activities.

In the eliminations to the outside we thus see the outcome of astrally oriented activity. And when materials incorporated in the elimination have been taken to the inorganic level the I organization also lives in them. And *this* life of the I organization does in fact have very special significance. For the energy used to effect such eliminations creates a counter-pressure going inwards, as it were. And this is essential for the healthy existence of the organism. Uric acid separated off in the urine creates the right inclination for sleep in the organism as such an inward counter-pressure. Too little uric acid in the urine and too much in the blood results in a period of sleep which is so short that it is not sufficient for the health of the organism.

13
On the Nature of Illness and Healing

Pain occurring somewhere in the organism is living experience in astral body and I. Both the astral body and the I are involved in the physical body and the etheric body in a specific way for as long as the human being is in the waking state. When sleep comes, the physical and the etheric body perform the organic activity on their own. The astral body and the I are then separate from them.

In sleep, the organism returns to the activities that came at the starting point of its development, in the embryonic period and early infancy. In the waking state, processes coming at the end of human development, processes of ageing and dying, predominate.

At the beginning of human development we have predominance of etheric body activity over astral body activity; the latter gradually increases in intensity, and etheric body activity moves into the background. In sleep the etheric body does not gain the intensity it had at the beginning of life. It continues at the intensity it developed relative to the astral in the course of life.

In every organ of the human body, the specific intensity of etheric activity allotted to it at every stage in life corresponds to a specific intensity of astral activity. It depends on the right relationship if the astral body is to be able to involve itself in the etheric body as appropriate or not. If it cannot do so because etheric activity is reduced, pain develops; if the etheric body develops a

level of activity that goes beyond the normal, interpenetration of astral and etheric activity becomes particularly intensive. This gives rise to pleasure, a feeling of
ease. We simply have to understand that beyond a certain level pleasure becomes pain, and conversely pain
becomes pleasure. If we ignore this, the above statement
might appear to contradict earlier statements.

An organ becomes diseased if the etheric activity
allotted to it cannot develop. Take metabolic activity, for
instance, which extends throughout the organism from
the digestive process. If the products of metabolism are
always completely converted to activity and substance
configuration in the organism, this is a sign that the
etheric body is functioning in the right way. If, however,
substances are deposited along metabolic pathways and
do not become part of the organism's activity, the ether
body's functionality is reduced. Physical processes normally stimulated by the astral body, but serving the
organism only within their sphere, go outside their own
sphere and enter into that of etheric activity. This gives
rise to processes that owe their existence to the predominance of the astral body. These processes have their
rightful place where ageing, involution of the organism,
occurs.

It is now a question of establishing harmony between
etheric and astral activity. The etheric body needs to be
strengthened, the astral body weakened. This may be
done by taking the physical substances which the ether
body processes to a level where they accept that activity
more easily than happens in the diseased state. The I
organization also needs to be given strength, for the
astral body, whose activity is oriented towards the animal, will be inhibited to a greater degree than otherwise if

the I organization is strengthened in the direction of human organization.

A way to penetrate these things perceptively will be found if we observe the activities some substance or other develops along the metabolic pathways. Take sulphur, for instance. It is found in protein. It therefore is the basis of the whole process which occurs when protein food is taken up. Sulphur proceeds from foreign etheric nature through the inorganic state to the etheric activity of the human organism. It is found in the fibrous matter of organs, in the brain, in nails and hair. It therefore passes along the metabolic pathways, going as far as the periphery of the organism. It proves to be a substance that plays a role in taking proteins into the sphere of the human ether body.

The question arises whether sulphur also has significance in the transition from the sphere of etheric activities to that of astral activities, and whether it has anything to do with the I organization. It does not noticeably combine with inorganic substances introduced into the body to form acids and salts. Such a compound would be the basis for taking sulphur processes into the astral body and I organization. Sulphur thus does not enter into these. It develops its activities in the sphere of the physical and the ether body. This is also evident from the fact that increased sulphur intake into the organism causes sensations of dizziness and reduced consciousness. Sleep, the state of the body in which astral body and I organization are not active as soul qualities, also becomes more intensive with increased sulphur intake.

We can see from this that sulphur given as a medicine makes the organism's physical activities more inclined to accept the intervention of etheric activities than they are in the diseased state.

The situation is different with phosphorus. It is found in the human organism as phosphoric acid and phosphates in protein, fibrous matter, in the brain, in the bones. It pushes in the direction of the inorganic substances that have significance in the sphere of the I organization. It stimulates conscious activity in man. It therefore brings about sleep in a way that is the opposite to that of sulphur, so that stimulation of conscious activity is followed by sleep; sulphur on the other hand brings about sleep by increasing unconscious physical and etheric activity. Phosphorus is present in the calcium phosphate of bones, which are organs subject to the I organization when it uses external mechanical activity to effect bodily movement, and not when it acts from within, in growth, regulation of metabolism, etc.

Phosphorus will therefore prove medicinal if the pathological condition consists in hypertrophy of the astral region over the I organization and the latter has to be strengthened so that the astral is pushed back.

Consider rickets. It has been said earlier on that it is due to hypertrophy of etheric and astral activity and leads to inadequate involvement of the I organization. If we first treat it with sulphur in a suitable way, etheric activity is strengthened relative to astral activity; if we let phosphorus treatment begin after this, the process we have been preparing in the ether organization is taken over into that of the 'I'; we thus counter rickets from two sides. (We know that phosphorus treatment for rickets has been put in doubt; however, the attempts at treatment made until now have *nothing* to do with the method described here.)

14
The Therapeutic Way of Thinking

Silica takes its actions along the metabolic pathways to the parts of the human organism where living matter becomes lifeless. It is found in the blood through which the configuring forces have to pass; and it occurs in hair, that is, at the point where configuration has its outer limit; you find it in bones, where configuration comes to its conclusion inwardly. It presents in urine as a product that has been separated off.

It provides the physical basis for the I organization. For this effects configuration. This I organization needs the silica process in the organism, all the way to the areas where configuration, the giving of form, borders on the outer and inner (unconscious) world. At the periphery of the organism, where the hair contains silica, the human organization is connected with the unconscious outside world. In the bones, this organization is connected with the unconscious inner world in which the will is active.

Between the two spheres of silica action, the physical basis of conscious awareness must develop in a healthy human organism. Silica has a twofold task. Inwardly it sets a limit to processes of pure growth, nutrition, etc. And on the outside it keeps purely natural processes away from the inner organism, so that the organism does not have to effect a continuation of natural processes but is able to develop its own.

In its youth, the human organism is provided with the highest levels of silica in areas where the tissues with configuring forces are located. From there silica evolves its activity in the direction of both border regions, creating a space between them where the organs of conscious life can develop. In a healthy organism these are predominantly the sense organs. But it has to be remembered that the life of the senses exists throughout the human organism. Interaction between the organs is based on the fact that one organ always perceives the activities of the other. In organs that are not sense organs in the true sense of the word, e.g. liver, spleen, kidney, etc., perception is so subtle that it remains below the threshold of conscious awareness in ordinary waking life. Apart from serving a specific function in the organism, every organ is also a sense organ.

The fact remains that the whole human organism is full of sensory perceptions that influence one another, and it has to be such in order that everything in it may work together in a healthy way.

All this bases on the right distribution of silica actions. We may actually speak of a silica organism incorporated in the organism as a whole; on it rests the sensitivity organs have for each other which is the basis for healthy vital functions, and it is also the basis for their right relationship to the inner life for the evolution of soul and spirit and to the outside so that natural processes are properly excluded.

This special organism will only function properly if the amount of silica present in the organism is such that the I organism is able to utilize it fully. If there is any additional silica, the astral organization, which is below the I organization, must be strong enough to eliminate it in the urine or in other ways.

Excess silica that has not been eliminated or taken

hold of by the I organization must be deposited as foreign matter in the organism and cause disruption for the I organization because of its tendency to configure, a tendency which actually serves that organization if it is present in the right amount. Too much silica introduced into the organism will therefore cause gastric and intestinal problems. It then is the task of the digestive sphere to eliminate a principle that is imposing excessive configuration. Drying out results where fluidity should prevail. This is above all evident when the soul's equilibrium is upset, with organic disturbances clearly perceptible in the background, due to excessive silica intake. Sensations of dizziness develop, the individual cannot prevent himself from falling into the sleep state, and finds that hearing and visual perception cannot be directed in the normal way; indeed, one may get the feeling that activities of the senses are being dammed up and unable to continue into the inner nervous system. All this shows that silica pushes towards the periphery of the body, but if too much of it gets there normal configuration is upset because there is a tendency to foreign configuration. The inner border of configuration is also upset. Problems are experienced in directing the locomotor system, joint pain. The whole may develop into inflammatory processes, which develop in areas where the foreign configuration tendency of silica comes in too strongly.

This indicates the medicinal powers silica is able to evolve in the human organism. Let us assume an organ that is not an actual sense organ becomes hypersensitive in its unconscious powers of perceiving parts of the organism that lie outside itself. You will note that the functions of this organ become abnormal. If you are in a position to give silica and correct the hypersensitivity this would be a way of dealing with the pathological condition. It will merely be a matter of influencing the organic bodily action to such effect that the silica which is introduced acts specifically around the diseased organ and does not have a systemic effect on the whole body in the sense described above.

By combining silica with other agents it is possible to arrange that the silica introduced into the body reaches exactly the organ where it is required and can be taken out of the body again from there as an elimination without causing harm to other organs.

A different situation occurs when the sensitivity of an organ for other organs is reduced. In that case, silica activity has cumulated in the periphery of the organ. It is then necessary to achieve such an influence on silica activity in the whole organism that the local activity loses its power, or one can use eliminators to encourage removal of the silica. The first method is preferable, as cumulation of silica in one site usually causes a deficit elsewhere. Distribution of localized silica activity over the whole organism can be achieved with a course of sulphur treatment, for example. You will realize why this is so if you read up on the sulphur actions in the organism elsewhere in this book.

15
The Method of Treatment

Insight into medicinal actions is based on gaining a full picture of the forces that evolve in the world outside man. For to initiate a healing process we must introduce substances into the organism that will spread in it in such a way that the pathological process gradually becomes a normal one. The nature of the pathological process is such, of course, that something occurs in the organism which does not become part of its total activity. This is something which such a process has in common with a process in the natural world outside.

We may say that disease develops when a process developing in the inner organism is similar to one in outside nature. Such a process may involve the physical or the etheric organism. Either the astral body or the I must then perform a function it does not usually perform. At a time of life when they should be coming into their own in independent activity of soul, they have to wind themselves back to an earlier period of life—in many cases actually the embryonic period—and become involved in the creation of physical and etheric configurations that should already exist in the sphere of the physical and the etheric organism; i.e. configurations taken care of by the astral body and the I organization in the earliest part of human life and later taken over by the physical and etheric organism only. For *all* development in the human organism depends on the principle that the total configuration of the physical and etheric body results originally from the activity of the astral and of the I organization; and that as life progresses astral and I activity continue in the physical and etheric organization. If they do not, the astral body and the I organization have to intervene in a way for which they are no longer suitable at this stage of their development.

Let us assume there is stasis in the lower abdomen. The physical and etheric organizations have failed to perform the functions they were given to perform in this part of the body in the preceding stage of life. Astral and I activity have to intervene. This weakens them for other functions in the organism. They are not where they should be, e.g. in the configuration of the nerves that go into the muscles. The result are signs of paralysis in some parts of the organism.

It is now a matter of introducing substances into the human organism that are able to relieve the astral and the I organization of activities that have not been allotted to them. You may find that the processes involved in creating powerful volatile oils in the plant organism, and specifically in the development of flowers, can thus relieve. Substances that contain phosphorus can also do it. All we have to do is take care to add other substances to the phosphorus so that its action develops in the intestine and not in metabolism that lies outside the intestine.

If there are inflammatory changes in the skin, astral body and I organization are developing abnormal activity in that part. They then withdraw from the functions they should perform in more internal organs. They reduce the sensitivity of internal organs. With their sensitivity reduced, these in turn cease to perform the processes assigned to them. The result may be abnormal conditions in liver function, for instance. And this may influence the digestion in the wrong way. If silica is introduced into the organism, the activities of the astral and the I organism on the skin are relieved. The inward-directed activity of these organisms is made available again; and a healing process sets in.

When we have pathological states that show themselves in palpitations, this is a case of irregular activity of the astral organism acting on the blood circulation process. This activity is then weakened with regard to brain processes. Epileptic states develop because reduced astral activity in the head organism puts too much of a strain on the etheric activity belonging to that area. If we introduce the gum-like substance that may be obtained from *Levisticum* (lovage)—in form of a tea, or even better processed to some degree to obtain a medicinal preparation—into the organism, the astral body activity that is wrongly applied to the blood circulation is released and made stronger in the brain organization.

In all these cases suitable diagnostic methods must determine the direction of the pathological actions. Take the last case. It may be that the original cause was disrupted interaction between etheric and astral body in the blood circulation. The cerebral signs are the consequence. Treatment may then be instituted in the way described.

The situation may be the other way round, however. The irregularity may originally have developed between the astral and the etheric activity in the cerebral system. In that case, irregular blood circulation and abnormal cardiac activity result. We then have to introduce sulphates into the metabolic process, for instance. The effect of these on the etheric organization of the brain is to cause a strong attraction to the astral body. We can observe this from the fact that thinking initiative, the sphere of the will and the whole integrity of the individual's nature show a change for the better. It will then probably prove necessary to support the astral forces, using a copper salt, for instance, so that they may grow into their new action on the circulatory system.

You will find that the total organism returns to its regular activity when excess activity caused by the astral and I organism in some part of the body is replaced by an activity brought about from outside. The organism has the tendency to balance its deficits. It will therefore restore itself if an irregularity is artificially regulated for a time to such effect that the process that has been provoked inside and which has to stop is fought with a similar process that is set in scene from without.

16
Perceiving Medicinal Qualities

Substances to be considered for medicinal use must first of all be known in such a way that their potential powers outside and inside the human organism can be assessed. Only to a minor degree would this be a question of considering the potential actions investigated by conventional chemists; what matters is to observe the actions that arise in the context of the inner constitution of forces a substance has in relation to the forces that radiate from the earth or into it.

Consider stibnite (grey antimony ore) from this point of view, for instance. Antimony relates strongly to the sulphur compounds of other metals. The sum total of sulphur properties remains constant within relatively narrow limits. It is sensitive to natural processes such as heating, combustion, etc. This also enables it to play a significant role in proteins, which separate completely from the earth forces and enter into the sphere of etheric actions. When antimony combines with sulphur on the basis of its affinity, it easily enters into the ether actions with it. It is thus easily introduced into protein activity in the human body, helping it to an ether action when, due to some pathological condition, the body is not itself able to transform a protein taken in from outside and make it part of its own activity.

But antimony also has other characteristics. Wherever possible it seeks to assume a configuration of radiating masses. It organizes itself along lines that go away from the earth and towards the forces active in the etheric. With antimony we therefore introduce something into the human organism that meets the action of the ether body half way. The process involved in antimony liquation also points to the relationship the substance has to the ether. It becomes finely fibrous in the process. Liquation is a process that may be said to start below, as something physical, and becomes etheric up above. Antimony makes itself part of this transition.

Antimony, which oxidizes on roasting, produces a white vapour on combustion that deposits on cold bodies to produce antimony bloom (valentinite).

Antimony also has some power to resist electrical actions. If treated in a certain way by electrolysis and made to precipitate at the cathode, the precipitate will explode if touched with a metal pointer.

All this shows that antimony has a tendency to enter *easily* into the ether element the moment conditions are even the least bit suitable. Seen with the eye of the spirit, all these details are mere pointers; for it has direct perception of the relationship between I activity and antimony actions, showing that antimony processes act like the I organization if introduced into the human organism.

In the human organism the blood shows a tendency to coagulate in its flow. This is the tendency which is under the influence of the I organization and has to be regulated under that influence. Blood is an intermediary organic product. Anything produced in the blood has gone through processes that are on the way to becoming processes of the full human organism, i.e. the I organization. It still has to go through processes that fit in with the configuration of this organism. The nature of these will be apparent from the following. By coagulating on removal from the body, blood shows that it has an inherent tendency to coagulation and has to be continually prevented from coagulating in the human organism. The principle which prevents blood from coagulating is the one through which the organism makes it part of itself. It becomes part of the body's configuration through the form-giving forces that come immediately prior to coagulation. If coagulation were to occur, life would be put at risk.

If we then have a pathological condition in the organism which consists in a deficit of the forces that go in the direction of blood coagulation, antimony in one form or another will prove medicinal.

The *configuration* of the organism is essentially a transformation of protein which causes it to work together with mineralizing forces. Such forces are found in calcareous matter, for instance. The point is beautifully illustrated in the development of the oyster shell. The oyster has to get rid of the shell-producing process in order to maintain the inherent nature of its protein. The situation is similar for the development of an egg shell.

In the oyster, calcareous matter is *separated off* so that it may *not* be incorporated in protein synthesis. In the human organism this incorporation has to take place. Mere protein activity has to be transformed into an activity involving the configuring forces evoked in calcareous matter by the I organization. This has to happen within blood production. Antimony counteracts the force that eliminates calcareous matter and because of its affinity with the ether element takes protein that wants to preserve its form into the state of formlessness that is receptive to the influences of calcareous and similar matter.

In the case of typhoid fever it is evident that the pathological condition consists in protein being insufficiently converted to blood substance capable of being configured. The type of diarrhoea which develops shows that inability to make this conversion actually begins in the intestine. The severe clouding of the conscious mind which develops shows that the I organization is driven out of the body and cannot take effect. The reason for this is that the protein cannot reach the mineralizing forces in which the I organization is able to be active. This view is also supported by the fact that evacuations are infectious. The tendency to destroy the configuring forces is enhanced in them.

Suitable compound antimony preparations used to treat typhoid symptoms prove medicinal. They strip the protein of its inherent forces and make it inclined to adapt to the configuring powers of the I organization.

People taking the widely held points of view of today will say that views like those outlined here for antimony are not exact; they will refer instead to the exact nature of accepted chemical methods. However, when it comes to actions in the human body, the chemical actions of substances have in fact as little relevance as the chemical composition of a pigment has for the way a painter uses it. Yes, it would be a good idea for a painter to know something about the chemical point of origin. But the way he *uses* pigments when he is painting is based on another methodology. The same applies to the medical practitioner. He may take chemistry as a basis that has some significance; but the mode of action substances have in the human organism no longer has anything to do with this chemical aspect. Anyone who holds the view that only data established in chemistry—and that includes pharmaceutics—are exact destroys the possibility of developing views on what happens when healing processes occur in the organism.

17
Perceiving the Nature of Substances as a Basis of Pharmacognosy

Anyone wishing to assess medicinal actions has to have an eye for the actions of forces that develop in the human organism when a substance which has specific actions outside the human organism is in some way or other introduced into it.

A classical example is given in the case of formic acid. It is a corrosive substance developed in the ant's body which causes inflammation. There it presents as a product that has been separated off. The animal organism in question has to produce this if it is to perform its functions in the right way. Life lies in separating-off activity. Once the separated-off material has been produced it has no further function in the organism. It has to be eliminated. The nature of the organism lies in what it does, not in its substances. The organization is not a complex of physical matter but an activity. Matter holds the stimulus for action within it. Once it has lost this stimulus it has no further significance for the organization.

The human organism also produces formic acid. There it has its significance. It serves the I organization. Through the astral body, parts of organic substance that go in the direction of becoming lifeless are separated out. The I organization needs this transition of organic substance to the lifeless state. But it is the process of transition it needs; not the product of the transition. Once matter going in the direction of becoming lifeless has been created it is a burden inside the organism. It either has to be separated off as it is, or dissolved and thus removed indirectly.

If the dissolution of something that should be dissolved fails to happen, the material cumulates in the organism where it may form the basis for gouty or rheumatic conditions. This is where the formic acid produced in the human organism comes into play as a solvent. If it is produced in adequate amounts, the organism will remove products going in the direction of lifelessness in the right way. If the power to produce it is reduced, gouty or rheumatic conditions develop. By introducing it into the organism from outside we support the organism, giving it what it is unable to produce itself.

We can get to know such modes of action if we compare one substance with another to see how it continues the action in the human organism. Take oxalic acid. Under certain conditions this converts to formic acid. The actions of the latter are a metamorphosis of oxalic acid. Oxalic acid is a secretion in the plant sphere, formic acid in the animal sphere. In the plant organism, oxalic acid develops an activity analogous to the production of formic acid in the animal. This means that oxalic acid production relates to the sphere of the etheric, formic acid production to the sphere of the astral. Diseases coming to expression in gouty and rheumatic conditions originate in inadequate astral body activity. Other conditions present in such a way that the causes, which in the case of gout and rheumatic conditions originate in the astral body, have been put back into the etheric organism. Then we have not only stasis of forces going in the astral direction, which presents an obstacle to the I organization, but also obstructive effects in the etheric that the astral organization is unable to overcome. These take the form of sluggish activity in the abdomen, inhibition of hepatic and splenic functions, stone-like deposits in the gall-bladder, and the like. If oxalic acid is given in such cases, we are suitably supporting the activities of the etheric organism. Oxalic acid effects a strengthening of the etheric body because the power of the I organization is transformed into a power of the astral body by the acid and the latter then has a stronger effect on the ether body.

Basing ourselves on observations of this kind, we can get to know the action of substances that prove medicinal in the organism. Observation may start with plant life. In the plant, physical activity is permeated with etheric activity. Here we can see what can be achieved by etheric activity. In the animal's astral organism, this activity becomes astral. If it is weak at the etheric level, adding the activity of an introduced plant product will strengthen it. The human organism has the animal principle as its basis. *Within certain limits*, the same applies to the interaction of human etheric and astral body as in the animal sphere.

It will be possible to restore the upset relationship between etheric and astral activity with medicines taken from the plant world. Such medicines will not serve our purpose, however, if some disorder exists in the way the physical, etheric and astral human organization interacts with the I organization. The I organization must direct its activities to processes that go in the direction of becoming mineral.

Only mineral principles will therefore prove medicinal for pathological conditions in this area. To get to know the medicinal actions of a mineral principle, we have to investigate a substance to see how it can be degraded. In the organism, mineral substance introduced from outside has to be degraded and recreated in a new form using our inherent organic forces. The medicinal action must consist in such degradation and recreation. The result of this must go in the direction that inadequate activity of the organism is taken over by the activity of the medicines which have been given.

Take excessive menstruation, for example. Here the power of the I organization has been weakened. It is one-sidedly utilized to generate blood. Too little remains of it for the blood absorptive power in the organism. The route which should be taken by forces going in the direction of the lifeless in the organism is too short, because these forces are too vehement. They become exhausted half-way along the road.

We come to their aid if we introduce some kind of calcium compound into the organism. This takes an active part in haemopoiesis. The I activity is relieved of this sphere and can turn to blood absorption.

18
Eurythmy Therapy

'Eurythmy therapy' plays a special role in our clinical approach.[3] It has been developed out of anthroposophy by Rudolf Steiner, initially as a new *art* form.

Its essential nature as eurythmic art has been frequently described by Rudolf Steiner, and it has already become widely known as an art.

On stage it presents the human being in movement; it is not a form of dance, however. Apart from anything else this is evident from the fact that it is mainly the arms and hands of the human beings that are in motion. Groups of people in motion elevate the whole to a stage presentation that is artistic in itself.

All movements are based on the inner nature of the human organization. Speech flows from this in the early years of human life. As speech sound wrests itself from the human constitution, so genuine insight into this constitution makes it possible to evolve movements from a single individual or a group of people that are *genuine* visible speech or visible song. These movements are no more arbitrary than the movements of speech. Just as we cannot pronounce an *O* in a word when there should be an *I* [as in mien], so an *I* or a *C sharp* can only be presented by one distinct gesture in eurythmy. Eurythmy is thus a genuine revelation of human nature that does not evolve from it unconsciously, the way speech or song may do, but can be consciously developed out of genuine insight into the nature of the human being.

In performances, you see individuals or groups of people in movement on the stage. The text, now translated into visible speech, is recited at the same time. You hear the content of the text and at the same time see it before your eyes. Or a musical item may be presented that reappears as visible song in movement and gestures.

Eurythmy presents, as sculpture in motion, a considerable extension to the sphere of the arts.

The discoveries thus made in form of an art can be developed in two directions. One is education. At the Waldorf School in Stuttgart, which was founded by Emil Molt and is guided by Rudolf Steiner, educational eurythmy is part of the curriculum for all classes, as well as physical training. The point is that the usual physical training only develops the dynamics and statics of the physical body. In eurythmy, the whole human being flows into the movement in body, soul and spirit. The developing young person is able to feel this, and will find these eurythmic exercises as natural, as an expression of human nature, as he would learning to speak in earlier years.

The other direction is in medicine. If the movements and gestures of eurythmy as an art and as used in education are modified so that they flow from the diseased nature of the human being just as the others do from a healthy nature, we have eurythmy therapy.

Movements made in this way have an effect on the organs affected by disease. We see how something done in an external way continues on to bring health to the organs, providing the gesture in motion exactly suits the pathological condition of the organ. This method of working on the body through movement addresses body, soul and spirit, and because of this it has a more intense influence on the inner human being in sickness than any other movement therapy.

This means, however, that eurythmy therapy can never be the business of lay people and must not be considered or treated as such.

A eurythmy therapist needs to be well trained in understanding the human organization and can only work in collaboration with a physician. Anything amateurish can only lead to trouble.

Proper diagnosis is the only basis for eurythmy therapy. The actual results seen with eurythmy therapy are such that it may indeed be called a blessing in the context of the clinical approach presented in these pages.

19
Characteristic Illnesses

In this chapter we present a number of case records from the Institute of Clinical Medicine in Arlesheim. They will show how the attempt may be made to use insights into the non-physical aspect of the human being in order to gain such a comprehensive picture of the pathological condition that diagnosis immediately shows which medicine needs to be used. The underlying approach sees falling ill and restoration to health as parts of the same cycle. Disease begins with an irregularity in the composition of the human organism as regards its aspects, which have been described in this book. It has reached a certain point by the time the patient comes for treatment. We need to see to it that all processes that have taken place in the human organism from the beginning of the disease go in reverse again, so that we finally arrive at the state of health the organism had before this. Such a process, which reverses on itself, cannot be achieved without a loss of growth forces in the total organism that is equal in value to the forces the human organism needs to grow in volume in its childhood. The medicines should therefore be such that they do not only reverse the pathological process but also support the patient's vitality, which is going down. Part of this latter effect will have to be left to the diet given to the patient. However, in more serious cases of illness the organism is not, as a rule, in a position to develop sufficient vitality in the processing of foods. It will therefore be necessary to make the actual treatment such that the organism is also given support in this direction. This has certainly been done with the typical medicines developed at the institutes of clinical medicine. It therefore needs fairly detailed study before one realizes why a preparation has certain constituents. In the evolution of the disease, attention must be paid not only to the localized disease process but to changes in the organism as a whole, which must be included in the process of reversal. How our thinking should go in the individual case will be shown by specific cases that we are going to characterize. Having described them, we shall continue with general considerations.

Case 1

This was a woman aged 26. The whole person showed an extraordinary degree of instability. The patient showed quite clearly that the part of her organism which we have called the astral body in this book was in a state of excessive activity. One saw that this astral body could not be adequately controlled by the I organization. If the patient wanted to do some work, the astral body immediately came to a boil. The I organization tried to make itself felt but was constantly repulsed. As a result the temperature goes up in such a case. In a healthy individual, regular digestive activity depends on the I organization functioning normally. Impotence of this I organization came to expression as persistent constipation in the patient. One consequence of this problem in the digestive system were the migraine-type conditions and vomiting she presented with. In sleep it is evident that the impotent I organization causes the organic activity that goes from below upwards to be inadequate, damaging exhalation. The result of this is excessive cumulation of carbon dioxide in the organism during sleep, which shows itself at the organic level as palpitations on waking, and on the psychological level in feelings of anxiety and shouting. Physical examination showed nothing but a deficit of the forces that effect a regular relationship between astral body, ether body and physical body. Excessive independent astral activity means that too few forces flow from the astral body to the physical and ether body. The latter therefore continue to be delicate in development during the growth period. On examination this was evident from the fact that the patient had a gracefully slender, weak body and complained of frequent back pain. Back pain develops because spinal marrow activity is exactly the site where the I organization must make itself felt most strongly. The patient also spoke of many dreams. This was due to the astral body evolving excessive independent activity when separated from the physical and ether body during sleep. As a first step, we had to strengthen the I organization and reduce astral activity. The first is achieved by selecting a medicine able to support the I organization where it is getting weak in the digestive tract. Copper may be recognized to be such a medicine. Used in form of a copper ointment dressing placed over the lumbar region, copper has a strengthening effect on inadequate warmth development which comes from the I organization. We shall see that abnormal cardiac activity is reduced and the feelings of anxiety disappear. Excessive independent activity of the astral body can be combated with minimal doses of lead taken by mouth. Lead pulls the astral body together and wakes the forces in it through which it combines more strongly with the physical body and the ether body. (Lead poisoning consists in the astral body being too strongly connected with the ether and physical body, so that the latter are subject to an excessive process of destruction.) The patient showed distinct improvement with this treatment. Her instability gave way to a certain inner firmness and certainty. Her state of mind changed from being torn apart to being inwardly contented. The symptoms of constipation and back pain disappeared, and so did the migraine-like conditions and headaches. The patient had her ability to work restored to her.

Case 2

Male patient aged 48; had been robust as a boy, psychologically sound. Stated that he was treated for nephritis for 5 months during the war and discharged fit. Married at age 35, five healthy children, a sixth died at birth. At age 33, mental overexertion was followed by depression, tiredness, apathy. These continued to get worse. Parallel to this he felt he had lost his bearings. He faced questions that revealed the negative sides of his work to him—he was a teacher—and he had nothing positive to set against this.—The pathological condition showed an astral body with too little affinity to the ether and physical body and immobile in itself. Because of this, the physical and ether body brought their own inherent qualities into play. The inner feeling of not being properly connected with the astral body caused depression; not being properly connected with the physical body tiredness and apathy. The way that the patient felt lost in spirit was due to the fact that the astral body was unable to utilize the physical and ether body. In connection with all this, sleep was good, because the astral body had little connection with the etheric and physical body. For the same reason, however, waking up was difficult. The astral body did not want to enter into the physical. A normal connection with the physical and ether body would only come in the evening, when they were tired. The patient therefore only really came awake in the evenings. The whole situation indicated that one had first of all to strengthen astral body activity. This can always be achieved by giving arsenic by mouth in form of a natural mineral water. You will find that after some time the individual has more control of his body. The connection between astral body and ether body grows stronger, depression, apathy and tiredness come to an end. Now it was also necessary to assist the physical body, which had grown sluggish in terms of movement because its connection with the astral body had been poor for a prolonged period, by giving phosphorus in minimal doses. Phosphorus supports the I organization, enabling it to overcome the resistance of the physical body. Rosemary baths open up a channel for the removal of deposited metabolic products. Eurythmy therapy will restore harmony between the different parts (system of nerves and senses, rhythmic system, motor and metabolic system) of the human organism when it has been upset by inactivity on the part of the astral body. If the patient is also given elder-flower tea, the sluggish metabolism which has gradually developed because of that inactivity on the part of the astral body will return to normal. We recorded a complete cure in the case of this patient.

Case 3

Male patient aged 31, artist, came to the clinic while on a concert tour in a condition of severe inflammatory functional disorder of the urinary organs; catarrhal symptoms, pyrexia, body excessively fatigued, general weakness, inability to work.

The history showed that the same condition had existed on a number of occasions before. Examination of his mental state showed a hypersensitive, worn-out astral body. A consequence of this was susceptibility of the physical and the ether body for catarrhal and inflammatory conditions. Even as a child, the patient's physical body had been rather weak, not well served by the astral body. Hence measles, scarlet fever, chickenpox, whooping cough, frequent sore throats; at age 14 urethritis, which recurred in conjunction with cystitis at age 29. At 18 he developed pneumonia and pleurisy; at 29, pleurisy again with an attack of influenza; at 30, frontal sinusitis. Persistent tendency to conjunctivitis.—His temperature initially was 38.9 °C during the two months he was an in-patient at the Clinic, and then went down, only to rise again on the 14th day; later it moved in waves between 37 and 36 °C, occasionally going up to above 37 °C, and would also go down to 35 °C. The temperature curve is a clear representation of variations of mood in the I organization. A curve of that type develops when the effects of half-conscious contents of the I organization become active in the warmth processes of the physical and etheric body, with the astral body failing to reduce them to a normal rhythm. The total action potential of the astral body was concentrated on the rhythmic system in this case, coming to expression in the giftedness of the artist. The other systems got less than their share. One important consequence was great tiredness and sleeplessness during the summer. In summer the astral body has many demands made on it by the outside world. Its inner action potential is reduced. The forces of the physical and ether body predominate. This presents as great tiredness in one's general feeling for life. The astral body's reduced action potential prevents it from separating from the physical body. This causes insomnia. Inadequate separation between astral body and ether body comes to expression in upsetting and unpleasant dreams which are due to sensitivity of this body to damage in the physical organism. Characteristically, the dreams symbolize this damage to the physical body in images of human mutilations. The terrifying aspect of these is the natural predominantly emotional content. One consequence of inadequate functioning of the astral body in the metabolic system is a tendency to chronic constipation. Independence on the part of the ether body, which is not sufficiently influenced by the astral body, means that proteins taken in with the food cannot be completely converted from vegetable and animal to human protein. Protein is thus eliminated in the urine, so that the protein test is positive. If the astral body does not function fully, processes foreign to the human organism develop in the physical body. The outcome of such processes is the development of pus. This represents a process in man that belongs to the outside world, as it were. The urinary sediment was found to contain pure pus, therefore. Pus formation has a psychological parallel. The astral body fails to process substances at the physical level and life's experiences at the psychological level. As matter is created as pus in a process that belongs outside the human being, soul contents arise that are outside the human range in character—an interest in abnormal situations in life, forebodings, omens, etc.— What we had to do was to bring balancing, cleansing and strengthening influences to bear on the astral body. The I organization being very active, its activity may be used as a vehicle, as it were, for the medicinal action. An I organization concentrated on the outside world is best treated by using medicinal actions that go inwards from outside. This is done by using compresses. We first of all put Melilotus on the compress. This acts on the astral body to distribute its forces and counteracts one-sided direction to the rhythmic system. It would, of course, be wrong to put the compresses on the part of the organism where the rhythmic system is specially concentrated. We put them around the organs where the metabolism and the motor system are concentrated. Head compresses were avoided because the change of mood in the I organization, which comes from the head, would inevitably inhibit the action. It was therefore a matter of encouraging the astral body and the I organization, which had to be put in harness together for the Melilotus action. This we sought to achieve by adding an oxalate taken from burdock root. The action of oxalic acid is such that I organization activity is changed into astral body activity. We also gave medicines in weak doses by mouth, designed to let separating-off processes become part of astral body functions in a regular way. We sought to normalize separating-off principles that were governed from the head organization by giving potassium sulphate. Potassium carbonate was given to influence processes depending on the metabolic system in the narrower sense. Teucrium was given to regulate the separating-off of urine. We therefore gave a preparation consisting of potassium sulphate, potassium carbonate and Teucrium. Throughout treatment account had to be taken of the highly unstable balance of the physical, psychic and spiritual organism as a whole. Continuous bed rest had to provide for physical equilibrium, peace of mind for mental equilibrium, and only this made it possible for the different medicines to work together. Movement and excitement would make the complex healing process almost impossible.—At the conclusion of treatment the patient was physically strong and vigorous, and in good condition mentally. It is clear that one disorder or another may recur if there is a further external attack of any kind, considering the unstable state of health. It is part of the whole healing process that attacks of this kind must be avoided in such a case.

Case 4

A child who had been brought to the Clinic twice, first at age 4, then at $5\frac{1}{2}$. Also its mother and the mother's sister. The process of diagnosis led from the child's illness to the mother's and also that of her sister. With the child, we found the following. It was a twin, born six weeks prematurely. The other child had died in the final embryonic stage. At the age of six weeks the child fell ill, crying a great deal, and was taken to hospital. Pylorospasm was diagnosed. The child was fed partly by a wet nurse, partly artificially. It was discharged from hospital at eight months. Arrived at home it had a seizure the first day, and this recurred daily for the first two months. The child would stiffen in an attack, turning up its eyes. Attacks were preceded by timidity and crying. The child also had a squint in the right eye and would vomit before an attack. At age $2\frac{1}{2}$ another attack occurred, lasting five hours. The child went stiff again and lay there as if dead. At age 4 it had an attack lasting 30 minutes. This was the first attack reported to be accompanied by pyrexia. The parents noted that the convulsions that happened after the child came back from hospital were followed by paralysis of the right arm and leg. The child made its first attempts at walking at age $2\frac{1}{2}$. It was only able to step out with the left leg, dragging the right leg after it. The right arm also remained without will impulses. The condition still persisted when the child was brought to see us. What we had to do was establish the situation with regard to the aspects of the child's organization. This was done independent of the syndrome. We found the ether body to be greatly atrophied, in some parts only accepting a very low level of astral body influence. The region of the right chest was as if paralysed in the ether body. On the other hand we noted something like a hypertrophy of the astral body in the stomach region. Then the syndrome had to be considered in relation to this. The astral body was clearly putting a considerable strain on the stomach in the digestive process, which, however, was static at the transition from intestine to lymph vessels because of paralysis of the ether body. This resulted in malnutrition of the blood. The symptoms of nausea and retching thus had to be taken very seriously. Seizures always result if the etheric body grows atrophic and the astral body comes to have a direct influence on the physical body, without mediation from the ether body. This applied very much in the case of this child. If the condition becomes permanent during the growth period, which was the case here, processes that make the motor system ready to receive the will in the normal way do not occur. This took the form of the child not being able to use the right side.—We then had to connect the child's condition with that of the mother. She was 37 years of age when she came to us. She stated that she had been as tall as she was now at age 13. Her teeth were bad at an early age, she had rheumatic fever as a child and maintained that she had had rickets. Menarche was relatively early. The patient said she had had a kidney disease at age 16, and also referred to some kind of seizures she had had. At age 25 she had chronic constipation because of spasms in the anal sphincter, which had to be stretched. She still had spasms with every stool.—Diagnosis of her condition, based on direct observation, with no conclusions drawn from her symptom complex, showed remarkable similarity with that of the child. Only everything was much milder in form. It had to be considered that the human ether body develops especially between the changing of the teeth and puberty. In the patient this was evident from the fact that the available forces of the ether body, which were not very strong, made growth possible only until she reached puberty. This is the point where the special development of the astral body began which, being hypertrophic, overwhelmed the ether body and intervened too strongly in the physical organization. This came to expression in cessation of growth at age 13. The patient was anything but dwarf size, however, and in fact very tall, which was due to the fact that the ether body's growth forces, uninhibited by the astral body, caused a tremendous increase in the volume of her physical body. These forces were not yet able at the time to intervene in the functions of the physical body in a regular way. This was evident in the development of rheumatic fever and later on of seizures. Because of weakness of the ether body, the action of the astral body on the physical body was particularly powerful. This was a destructive effect. In a normally developing life it is balanced out by constructive forces during sleep, when the astral body has separated from the physical and ether body. If the ether body is too weak, as in the case of our patient, excessive destruction occurs, and in her case this could be seen from the fact that she needed her first filling in her teeth in her 12th year. If the ether body has extra demands made on it, as in pregnancy, this will always cause dental deterioration. The weakness of the ether body as far as its connection with the astral body was concerned was also particularly evident in the frequency of dreams and in the fact that the patient slept soundly, despite all the irregularities. The weakness of the ether body was also apparent from the fact that foreign processes not controlled by the ether body occurred in the physical body, presenting as proteins, occasional hyaline casts and salts in her urine.—It is interesting to note the way these pathological processes relate to those of the mother's sister. The diagnosis concerning the composition of the aspects of the human being is almost entirely the same. Weak ether body activity, therefore dominance of the astral body. Only in her case the astral body itself is weaker than her sister's. Menarche was therefore early, too, but instead of inflammations she merely had pain due to irritation of the organs, e.g. the joints. The ether body has to be especially active in the joints if vitality is to go normally. If ether body activity is weak the activity of the physical body becomes dominant, which showed in swellings and chronic arthritis in this case. The weakness of the astral body, which is not acting sufficiently on subjective feelings, is evident from a preference for sweet foods, which increase sensation for the astral body. If in addition daily life has worn out a weak astral body, the pain will be more significant if the weakness persists. The patient complained of pain getting worse in the evenings.—The connection between the disease states of the three patients pointed to the generation ascendant to the two sisters, and especially the child's grandmother. The cause must lie with her. The upset balance between astral and ether body in all three patients can only have arisen from an equal imbalance in the child's grandmother. This irregularity must go back to the grandmother's astral and ether body not achieving adequate nutrition of the foetal membranes which feed the embryo, especially the allantois. This inadequate development of the allantois has to be looked for in all three patients. We established it first of all by purely spiritual methods. The physical allantois is metamorphosed, becoming non-physical, into the capability of the astral body's forces. A degenerated allantois results in reduced capability of the astral body, which shows itself especially in all motor organs. All this held true for all three patients. It is indeed possible to perceive the quality of the allantois by considering that of the astral body. It will be evident from this that our reference to the ascendance does not derive from hazardous conclusions based on fantasy but from genuine observations using the methods developed in the science of the spirit.

To anyone who feels irritated by this truth we would say that the above has nothing to do with a love for going against accepted views but a desire not to withhold insights, which after all have been gained, from anyone.

The mystical concepts of heredity will remain for ever obscure if we shy away from accepting the idea of metamorphosis from physical to non-physical and the reverse in the sequence of generations.

As regards treatment, an insight like the above must inevitably give us an idea as to where the healing process should be initiated. If we had not been pointed in the direction of the hereditary aspect but had merely noted the irregularity in the relationship between ether body and astral body, we would have used medicines that act on these two aspects of the human being. In the present case this would have proved ineffective, however, for the damage, going through generations, lies too deep to be balanced out in these aspects of the human organization themselves. In a case like this we have to influence the I organization, bringing everything into play that has to do with harmonizing and strengthening of the ether and astral body. We achieve this by addressing the I organization in enhanced sensory stimuli, as it were (sensory stimuli act on the I organization).—We attempted to do this in the following way for the child. A 5% pyrites ointment dressing was applied to the right hand and at the same time golden agaric ointment (*Amanita caesarea*) was massaged into the left half of the head. Externally applied, pyrites, an iron sulphide, stimulates the I organization to make the astral body more lively and increase its affinity to the ether body. The action of golden agaric substance, with organized nitrogen a special constituent, is to let an action going via the I organization evolve from the head that makes the ether body more lively and increases its affinity to the astral body. The healing process was supported by eurythmy therapy, which makes the I organization as such lively and active. This results in externally applied principles being taken to the depths of the organization. The healing process thus initiated was further enhanced by measures designed to make astral and ether body particularly sensitive to the influence of the I organization. Using a rhythmic diurnal sequence, baths were given with a decoction of Solidago, back rubs with a decoction of Stellaria media, and both a tea made of willow bark (acts specifically on the astral body's receptivity) and Stannum 0.001 (specifically makes the ether body receptive) by mouth. We also gave poppy juice in weak doses, to induce the individual's damaged inherent organization to make room for the medicinal actions.

The mother had more of the last of the above treatments, since she was one generation earlier so that hereditary forces were less involved. The same applied to the mother's sister.—We were able to note that while still at the Clinic the child was more biddable and the general psychological condition had improved. It was more obedient, for instance; and movements that had been very clumsy were done in a more skilful way. Later the aunt reported that the child had gone through a big change. It had become quieter, the excess of involuntary movements was reduced; it has gained sufficient skills to be able to play on its own; and, with reference to the psychology, its former obstinacy had disappeared.

Case 5

A woman aged 26 came to the Clinic suffering from serious consequences of an attack of influenza in 1918

in conjunction with pulmonary catarrh that had followed a pleurisy she had had in 1917. The patient had
never been really well since she had the influenza. In
1920 she was greatly emaciated, weak, with a slight
temperature and night sweats. Soon after the attack of
influenza she developed low back pain, which got
worse and worse until late in 1920; then the pain was
extremely severe and a curvature was noted in the
sacral region. Her right index finger became swollen.
Bed rest was stated to improve the back pain.—When
the patient came to us she had a congestive abscess in
the right thigh, bloated abdomen with slight ascites,
and catarrhal sounds over the apices of both the left
and the right lung. Digestion and appetite were good.
The urine was concentrated, with traces of protein.
Investigation using the science of the spirit showed
hypersensitivity of the astral body and the I organization; this kind of abnormality initially comes to expression in the ether body in that it does not develop
proper ether functions but an etheric offprint of the
astral functions. Astral functions are destructive.
Vitality and the normal process in the physical organs
therefore had to show atrophy. This is always connected with processes that are normally outside the
human being, as it were, taking place within the human
organism. The congestive abscess, the back pain, the
bloated abdomen, the catarrhal symptoms in the lung,
and inadequate processing of protein were due to
this.—Treatment had to consist in reducing the sensitivity of the astral body and the I organization. This is
done by giving silica, which always increases the
inherent powers to counter sensitivity. In this case we
added powdered silica to the food and gave it in

enemas. We also derived the sensitivity by putting mustard plasters on the lower back. The action of this is to generate sensitivity on its own accord, which relieves the astral body and I organization of sensitivity. A process to reduce astral body sensitivity in the digestive tract was used to channel this astral activity to the ether body, which is where it normally should be. This was achieved with copper and Carbo animalis in low doses. The possibility of the ether body refusing to take up normal digestive activity, having become unused to this, was countered by giving pancreatic juice.

The congestive abscess was aspirated a number of times. This removed large quantities of pus. The abscess was reduced and the abdominal swelling decreased, with pus formation decreasing steadily and finally ceasing. When pus was still being discharged, a further elevation of temperature took us by surprise one day. It did not seem inexplicable—for the constitution of the astral body being as described, even minor mental upsets could cause such a fever. Distinction must be made, however, between the explicable nature of such a fever and the severe damage it can cause. Under the given conditions, such a fever actually mediates profound intervention of destructive processes in the organism. Care must be taken immediately to strengthen the ether body, so that it will inhibit the damaging effect of the astral body. We used silver injections in high potency and this resulted in the temperature being reduced.— The patient had gained 10 kg in weight when she left the Clinic and was much stronger. We are perfectly aware that in this case follow-up treatment will be needed to reinforce the cure.

Incidental remark

The cases discussed so far were presented to characterize the principles we use to find the indicated medicines in the process of diagnosis. To illustrate this clearly we chose cases where treatment had to be highly individual. We have also produced typical medicines, however, that can be used to treat typical diseases. The case histories that follow show the use of such typical medicines.

Case 6. Treatment of hay fever

We had a patient with severe hay fever symptoms. He had been suffering with this from childhood. He came to us for treatment in his 40th year. For this condition we have our Gencydo preparation. It was given to the patient at the time—this was in May—when the disease was most acute. We treated him with injections and locally by painting the inside of the nose with Gencydo liquid. When there had been definite improvement at a time when the patient would still have been greatly troubled by his hay fever symptoms in earlier years, he went on a trip and was able to report that he was incomparably better compared to previous years. The next year he was again travelling from America to Europe during the hay fever season and had only one attack, much milder than before. Repeating the treatment resulted in a perfectly tolerable state for that year. To effect a thorough cure, the treatment was again repeated the following year, though there was no actual attack. The patient's own words in describing his condition for a further year were: 'In the spring of 1923 I resumed treatment because I expected further attacks. I found that my nasal mucosa was much less sensitive than before. My work necessitated my being in the midst of flowering grasses and pollen-producing trees. I also rode on hot and dusty roads all through the summer. But with the exception of one single day there were no hay fever symptoms for the whole summer; indeed I have every reason to believe that this one day only brought a cold and not an attack of hay fever. After 35 years this was the first year I was able to be and work freely in an environment where I truly went through hell in earlier years.'

Case 7. Treatment of sclerosis

A woman aged 61 presented at the Clinic with sclerosis and proteinuria. Her presenting condition had followed influenza with a slight temperature and gastrointestinal upset. She had not felt well since the attack of influenza. She complained of dyspnoea on waking, bouts of vertigo, and of a pounding sensation in head, ears and hands that was a particular problem on waking up but would also develop on walking and going up anything. Sleep was good. There was a tendency to chronic constipation, and protein in the urine. Blood pressure was 185 mmHg. First of all we considered the sclerosis, which was noticeable from hyperactivity of the astral body. The physical body and the ether body were unable to take in the whole activity of the astral body. In such a situation an excess of astral hyperactivity is not absorbed by the physical and ether body. Normal, firm maintenance of the human organization is only possible if absorption is complete. If this is not the case, the non-absorbed part makes itself felt in vertigo and, above all, subjective sensory illusions such as pounding, etc. The non-absorbed part also takes hold of ingested substances and imposes processes on them before they have entered into normal metabolism. This was evident in the tendency to constipation and elimination of protein; also in the gastrointestinal problems. Blood pressure is elevated in such cases because hyperactivity of the astral body also elevates I activity, which comes to expression in raised blood pressure.—We mainly treated this patient with our Scleron; we merely added Belladonna in very low dosage to support this and also deal with the vertigo at the time. We used elderflower tea to help the digestion, regulated her stools with enemas and laxative tea, and prescribed a salt-free diet because salts promote sclerosis. We saw relatively rapid improvement. The attacks of vertigo regressed, as did the pounding. The blood pressure went down to 112. Subjective improvement was rapid. The sclerosis did not advance in the year that followed. A year later the patient returned, with her symptoms less than before. Similar treatment brought further improvement; and now, some time since the treatment was given, it is clearly evident when seeing the patient that the sclerosis is not causing further degeneration of the organism. The outer symptoms characteristic of sclerosis are regressing and the rapid ageing to which the patient had previously been subject is no longer happening.

Case 8. Treatment of goitre

A woman who came to see us in her 34th year. She was the type of person whose whole mental makeup was strongly influenced by some degree of heaviness and inner brittleness of the physical body. It seemed as if every word she said was an effort. The concave nature of the face as a whole was highly characteristic; the root of the nose was like something held back in the organism. The patient stated that she had been delicate and sickly since her schooldays. As to actual diseases, she had only had a mild form of measles. She was always pale, and always much tired, with a poor appetite. She was sent on from one physician to another, with the following diagnoses made one after the other: pulmonary apicitis, gastritis, anaemia. To her own mind the patient felt she was not so much sick in body but more in soul.

Having given the history, let us refer to the spiritual-scientific diagnosis, so that we may then check everything against this.

The patient showed high-degree atony of the astral body. This held the I organization back from the physical and ether body. The whole of her conscious life was as though filled with a slight, dim sleepiness. The physical body was exposed to the processes deriving from the substances introduced into the body. As a result, these substances were converted into parts of the human organization. The coherent vitality of ether body was excessively subdued by the I and the astral body, which means that the inner responses of general feeling for life and the sensation of bodily statics grew much too lively, the agility of the outer senses much too dull. All bodily functions therefore had to take a course that caused them to be out of harmony with each other. It was inevitable that the patient would have the feeling she could not hold the functions of her body together with the I. This felt like psychic impotence to her. Because of this, she said she was more sick in soul than in body. With increasing impotence of the I and astral body, pathological conditions had to develop in the different parts of the body, which was also evident from the different diagnoses. Impotence of the I came to expression in irregularities in glands such as the thyroid and adrenals; also in irregularities in the gastrointestinal system. All this had to be expected in the case of this patient and could indeed be established. Her goitre and the condition of the gastrointestinal system were wholly in accord with the spiritual-scientific diagnosis. The following is highly characteristic. Because of impotence of the I and the astral body, part of the need for sleep was met during waking hours, with the result that her sleep was much less deep than that of normal people. This was experienced as persistent insomnia by the patient. In connection with this she had the feeling that she would go to sleep easily and wake up easily. Also in connection with this she thought she had numerous dreams, which however were not real dreams but mixtures of dreams and waking impressions. They were not remembered, therefore, and did not touch her deeply because the strength of the stimulus was reduced. In the internal organs the impotence of the I came to expression primarily in the lungs. Pulmonary apicitis is really always indicative of a weak I organization. The fact that the I did not take metabolism to its completion was revealed in rheumatic symptoms. Menarche was at age 14; the weak I organization did not provide sufficient development of strength to gear the menstrual process down again once it had got going. The work of the I in this gearing down process comes to conscious awareness through the nerves that enter the spinal cord in the sacral region. Pain is felt in nerves if the currents of the I organization and the astral body do not pass through them sufficiently. The patient complained of low back pain during her periods. All this showed the way to treatment as follows. We have found that Colchicum autumnale acts as a powerful stimulant on the astral body, specifically the part corresponding to the neck and head organization. Colchicum autumnale is therefore used by us to treat all diseases where goitre is the outstanding symptom. We therefore gave the patient 5 drops of our Colchicum preparation three times daily, and the goitre reduced in size with this and the patient felt relieved. Once we have strengthened the astral body in this way it also mediates a better function of the I organization, and medicines with potential actions on the digestive and reproductive organs are then able to take effect in the organism. We used wormwood enemas for this purpose, mixing them with oil because oil acts as an excitant in the digestive tract. We saw significant improvement with this medicine. We believe this treatment can prove particularly effective around the 35th year of human life as this is the time when the I organization has a marked affinity to the rest of the organism and is easily stimulated if weak. The patient was 34 when she came to us.

Case 9. Migraine-type states in the menopause

The patient came to us when she was 55. She stated that she had been a delicate, weak child; apparently she had measles, scarlet fever, chickenpox, whooping cough and mumps in her childhood. Menarche was at age 14-15. Menses were very strong and painful from the beginning.

In her 40th year she had a total hysterectomy because of a pelvic tumour. The patient also stated that from her 35th year she had had three-day episodes of migraine-type headaches every three or four weeks which developed into a disease affecting the head lasting three days, with unconsciousness in her 46th year.—The current spiritual-scientific diagnosis was: general weakness of the I organization coming to expression in the activity of the ether body not being sufficiently inhibited by the I organization. This resulted in vegetative organic functions spreading to the head and system of nerves and senses, something which does not reach that level if the I organization is normal. Certain symptoms were in accord with this diagnosis. The first was frequent urgency of micturition. This was due to the fact that the normally developed astral body, which regulates elimination via the kidneys, was not opposed by a sufficiently strong I organization which would normally restrain it. A second symptom was that she went to sleep late and woke up tired. Once she had woken up, the vital activity deriving from sleep which continues to take effect was experienced as fatigue because of the weak I. A third symptom was that she dreamt little. The I organization only imprinted faint images on the astral body and these could not come to expression in lively dreams.

These insights led us to initiate treatment as follows. We had to clear the I organization's way to the physical and ether body. We did this with sorrel salt (acid potassium oxalate) compresses on the forehead at night and compresses with 7% Urtica dioica solution on the lower abdomen in the mornings, with a 20% lime blossom solution on the feet at midday. The aim was to reduce vital activity during the night; the oxalate, which in the organism has the function of suppressing excessive vital activity, achieved this. In the mornings we had to see to it that the I organization found its way into the physical body. This was done by stimulating the circulation. The iron activity in the nettle was used for this purpose. It remained to encourage the penetration of the physical body with the I organization in the course of the day. This was done by utilizing the derivative, drawing effect of the lime blossom used at midday. The headaches which we have described had become more severe when the patient was in her 46th year. We had to connect these headaches with the cessation of her periods following the total hysterectomy, and [see] their worsening, with loss of consciousness, as a symptom of compensation for the menopause. We first attempted to improve this by using antimony. It should have given improvement if it had been a matter of general metabolism, which is regulated by the I organization. No improvement was achieved. This proved that it was a matter of the relatively independent part of the I organization that regulates mainly the reproductive organs. In our view, the root of Potentilla tormentilla given in high dilutions should be the specific in this case, and it did indeed prove effective.

20
Typical Medicines

Introductory remark

Below, a number of typical medicines we have partly put on the market will be described to show their medicinal value. They are designed for the treatment of typical diseases, and where typical aspects show themselves in a pathological state, our medicine must prove therapeutic in terms of what is presented in this book. A number of our medicines will be described from this point of view.

20.1 Scleron

This consists of metallic lead, honey and sugar. The action of lead on the organism is such that it encourages the destructive effects of the I organization. If it is therefore introduced into an organism where the destructive effect of the I organization is too little, encouragement results providing the dosage is high enough. If the dose is too strong, hypertrophy of the I organization occurs. The body destroys more than it creates and must fall into decay. In sclerosis the I organization is too weak; it does not itself show adequate destructive activity. Destruction is therefore effected by the astral body only. The products of degradation drop out of the organism and give extra strength to the organs which consist of salt substances. Lead in suitable doses restores destructive function to the I organization. The products of degradation do not remain in the body and cause hardening but are ejected. With sclerosis the only possible way of effecting a cure is to open a channel to the outside for the salt-forming processes that otherwise remain in the body. With lead we have given the processes of the I organization *direction*. It is also necessary to keep these processes volatile, as it were. This is done by adding honey. Honey enables the I organization to have proper control of the astral body. It thus removes the relative autonomy the astral body has in sclerosis. Sugar acts directly on the I organization. It strengthens it in itself. Our medicine therefore achieves the following. Lead has a destructive action like that of the I organization and not like the astral body. Honey conveys the destructive activity of the astral body to the I organization, and the sugar enables the I organization to perform its specific function.—It may be noted that the initial stages of sclerosis are evident from the fact that acuity of thought and exact control of memory cease. If our medicine is used at this early stage, it will be possible to avoid the more mature stages of sclerosis. It does, however, also prove effective at those later stages. (Directions for use are given on the label.)

20.2 Bidor for migraine

The head organization is such that the inner, greyish-white part of the brain is physically the most advanced part of the human organization. It contains sensory activity in which all the other senses are brought together, with the I and the astral body acting into this.

It takes an interest in the rhythmic system of the organism, which is influenced by the astral body and the ether body, and it also takes an interest, though only to a very slight degree, in the system of metabolism and limbs, which is influenced by the physical and ether body. This part of the brain differs from the peripheral brain enclosing it, which in its physical organization contains much more of the system of metabolism and limbs, a little more of the rhythmic system, but least of all of the system of nerves and senses. Migraine develops if an activity of the I organization has been knocked back, so that the central brain has less neurosensory activity and more digestive activity, i.e. gets more similar to the peripheral brain than it normally is. Its cure will therefore depend 1) on stimulation of neurosensory activity; 2) on a transformation of rhythmic activity from being inclined towards metabolism to being inclined towards respiration; 3) on limiting the purely vital metabolic activity that lacks regulation by the I organization. The first is achieved with silica. Silicon combined with oxygen contains processes that are like those which occur in the organism at the transition from respiratory to neurosensory activity. The second is achieved with *sulphur*. This contains the process by which the rhythm inclined towards the digestive system is changed into one inclined towards respiration. And the third is achieved with *iron*, which immediately after the digestive process of digestion channels metabolism into the process of the blood rhythm, which suppresses the metabolic process itself. Suitably processed *iron*, *sulphur* and *silica* must therefore be a medicine for migraine. We have found this confirmed in countless cases.

20.3 Pyrites for tracheitis and bronchitis

We will now discuss a medicament that owes its existence to insight capable of establishing the right relationship of processes of substances to processes in the human organism. It has to be taken into account that a substance really is a process brought to a halt, a frozen process as it were. We really should not speak of pyrites but of the pyrites process. This process, held fast as though frozen in the mineral pyrites, is something that can arise when the iron process and the sulphur process act together. Iron stimulates the blood circulation, as mentioned in the section on Bidor, and sulphur mediates the connection between blood circulation and respiration. The origin of tracheitis and bronchitis, and also of some forms of stammer, lies in the very place where blood circulation and respiration enter into a relationship. This process between blood circulation and respiration, which is also the process out of which the organs concerned are developed in embryonic life and continue to be renewed as life goes on, can be taken over by iron sulphur substance introduced into the body when it does not take its normal course in the organism. Based on this insight, we produce a medicament for the above pathology from pyrites, reconfiguring the mineral in such a way that its forces find their way into the affected organs when there is an internal indication. It is, of course, necessary to know the route particular substance processes take in the organism. The iron process is taken as far as the blood circulation by metabolism. The sulphur process moves from the blood circulation into the breathing process.

20.4 Actions of antimony compounds

Antimony has an extraordinarily powerful connection with other solids, e.g. sulphur. It thus shows us that it can easily follow the route which sulphur takes in the organism, e.g. to all respiratory processes. Another property of antimony is that it tends to crystallize in radiating masses. It thus shows us that it easily follows specific energy radiations in the earth's environment. This property is even more evident if antimony is subjected to the process of liquation. This makes it finely fibrous. And it shows itself even more significantly if antimony is taken through a combustion process and its white vapour develops. This vapour deposits on cold solids to produce the characteristic antimony bloom. Just as antimony follows the forces acting on it when outside the human organism, so it follows the form-generating forces when in the human organism. In the blood we have, as it were, a state of balance between form-generating and form-dissolving forces. Antimony is able, because of the above-mentioned properties, to take the form-generating forces of the human organism into the blood, providing the way is prepared through combination with sulphur. The powers of antimony are thus the ones at work in the coagulation of the blood. In terms of the science of the spirit, the situation is that the astral body is strengthened in the powers that lead to coagulation of the blood. One has to see forces similar to those of antimony in the astral body that act centrifugally from the inside to the outside. Against these antimonizing forces act the forces that go from the outside to the inside, liquefying the blood and putting liquefied blood as a plastic principle at the service of body development. The forces of protein also work in this direction. The forces contained in the protein process continually prevent the coagulation of the blood. Take the case of typhoid fever; it is a preponderance of albuminizing forces. By introducing antimony into the organism in extremely subtle doses, one acts against the forces that create typhoid fever. It must be taken into account, however, that the action of antimony is very different, depending on whether it is used internally or externally. With external application, in ointments and the like, it weakens the centrifugal forces of the astral body that come to expression in eczematous changes, for instance; with internal use it opposes the forces that are too powerfully centripetal, as seen in the case of typhoid fever.

Antimony is an important medicament in all conditions where consciousness is dimmed to a dangerous degree (somnolence). In this case, the form-giving, centrifugal forces of the astral body and hence the brain and sensory processes have been partly put out of action. If antimony is introduced into the organism, the missing astral forces are artificially created. It will always be found that taking antimony strengthens memory, enhances the creative powers of the soul and makes the state of soul more complete in itself. The organism is regenerated in a process that comes from the strengthened soul. An awareness of this existed in earlier times in medicine. Antimony was therefore a universal remedy for physicians of old. We may not take such an extreme position, but in view of the above we must nevertheless seek to consider antimony as a medicine that has many uses.

20.5 Cinnabar

We were able to perceive cinnabar to be an important medicinal agent. This is a substance where we have the opportunity to study the relationship of mercury to the human organism, a relationship that has been defended by many and challenged by many. Mercury is the frozen process which is right in the midst of the regenerative processes that within the organism separate the organism's essential nature off almost completely from itself. The mercury forces characteristically cause these separated-off forces to be absorbed again in the whole organism. Mercury may thus be clinically used (in extremely subtle doses) where processes develop in the organism that separate themselves from it and need to be brought under the control of the organism as a whole again. These are all catarrhal processes. They develop when external influences cause some tract of the organism to be wrested away from the control of the organism as a whole. This is the case with tracheitis and all catarrhal changes in that area. Mercury forces are medicinal if directed towards them. One property of sulphur that has been mentioned a number of times is that it is effective in the area of the organism where circulation and respiration meet, that is, in everything that comes from the lung. Cinnabar is a compound of mercury and sulphur; it is an effective medicament for all catarrhal changes in the above-mentioned areas of the human organism.

20.6 Gencydo as a hay fever medicine

The symptoms of hay fever are inflammatory changes in the mucosa of eyes, nose, throat and upper respiratory passages. The history of patients suffering from hay fever often shows that disease processes coming under the heading of 'exudative diathesis' occurred also in child-hood.—This points to the ether body and the way the astral body behaves. The forces of the ether body pre-ponderate, and the astral body withdraws, showing a tendency not to intervene properly in the etheric and physical body. Catarrhal symptoms arise when the orderly intervention of the astral body—and hence also the I organization—in the affected areas is disturbed. Astral body and I organization become hypersensitive, and this also explains the spasmodic attacks of reactions to sensory impressions such as light, heat, cold, dust and the like.—The healing process must therefore address the astral body, helping it to intervene in the proper way in the etheric body. This is possible if we use fruit juice from fruits with leathery skins. It is immediately apparent if one looks at these fruits that configuring principles act-ing inwards from the outside are particularly active in them. Giving such juices internally and applying then externally we achieve stimulation of the astral body in a direction going towards the ether body; their mineral constituents such as potassium, calcium and silica will at the same time cause support to be given by the I orga-nization (see chapter 17), so that one achieves genuine healing of the hay fever.—Detailed directions for use are included with the product.

Notes

1 Steiner, R., *Knowledge of the Higher Worlds, How is it Achieved?* (GA 10). Tr. D. S. Osmond, C. Davy. London: Rudolf Steiner Press 1976.
2 Dubois-Reymond, Emil (1818–1896), Berlin physiologist. The passage quoted was taken from 'Über die Grenzen des Naturerkennens. Ein Vortrag in der zweiten öffentlichen Stizung der 45. Versammlung deutscher Naturforscher und Ärzte zu Leipzig am 14. August 1872', Leipzig 1872, S. 25–27.
3 Steiner, R. *Curative Eurythmy* (GA 315). Tr. K. Krohn. Lecture of 29 October 1922. London: Rudolf Steiner Press 1983.

Earlier editions

Below are the Preface and Postscript Dr Wegman wrote for the earlier editions of this work.

Preface to the first edition

Our teacher, leader and friend Rudolf Steiner is no longer among the living. A serious illness, which arose from physical exhaustion, has taken him from us. He had to take to his bed when still fully engaged in his work, and his energies, which he had given in such great measure, never holding back, to his work in the Anthroposophical Society, were no longer sufficient to overcome the illness. All who loved and revered him had to experience, in great pain, that this human being, someone who had been able to help so many people, had to let destiny take its course where he himself was concerned, knowing full well that higher powers prevailed in this case.

The fruit of our common efforts is presented in this small volume.

The teachings of anthroposophy, which for medical science in particular is a gold mine of new ideas, were something I, as a physician, could fully accept, finding in them a source of wisdom on which it was possible to draw ever and always, and which can illumine and solve many problems that are still unsolved today. And so active cooperation developed between Rudolf Steiner and myself, deepening to such a degree, especially in the last two years, that it proved possible to write and produce a book between us. It had always been Rudolf Steiner's desire—and I was able to understand this fully—to renew the mysteries of old and let them enter into medicine. For those mysteries have from time immemorial been closely connected with the skills of healing, with the gaining of spiritual insights considered important in healing work. The aim was not to underestimate scientific medicine in an amateurish way; it was given full recognition. But it was important to add to existing knowledge the insights that can come from true perception of the spirit, enabling us to understand the processes of illness and healing. Of course the intention was not to bring the inward, instinctive ways of the ancient mysteries back to life, but to find a way that was in accord with the fully developed modern conscious mind, taking it up into the sphere of the spirit.

Thus a beginning was made, and the Institute of Clinical Medicine I had established in Arlesheim provided the practical background for the theories presented in this book. And we sought to show ways in the art of healing that seek to find an extension of medical knowledge along the lines indicated here.

We intended to follow this small volume with many things arising from our common work. Sadly this was no longer possible. I intend, however, to follow this volume with a second, perhaps even a third, based on the many suggestions and notes in my possession. — May this first volume, the manuscript of which was corrected by Rudolf Steiner with pleasure and inner satisfaction just three days before his death, find its way to all who seek to find a way from the riddles of life to an understanding of life in its glory and greatness.

Arlesheim-Dornach, September 1925

Ita Wegman, MD

Postscript

Up to this point we have had the fruit of our shared work, and, surely much regretted by all of us, writing had to cease when Rudolf Steiner's illness began. The plan had been to discuss in the continuation the earthly and cosmic forces active in the metals gold, silver, lead, iron, copper, mercury and tin, and to consider how they may be used in medicine. We also intended to show the deep insights people possessed in the ancient mysteries into the relationships between these metals and the planets, and their relationships to the different organs in the human organism. The intention was to speak of this knowledge and give it a new foundation.—My work in the immediate future will be to let the second part of the book appear soon, based on suggestions made to me and on my notes.

Editorial notes (from the publishers of the German in Dornach)

The present edition
Origin: 1st edition, 1925.
    From the 7th German edition (1991) onwards, the text

was compared with the first edition and corrected as required. Editorial changes made in the text compared to the first edition are listed below.

This book was written by Rudolf Steiner and Ita Wegman. Chapters 1–18 are in Rudolf Steiner's handwriting, chapters 19 and 20 in Ita Wegman's. The manuscript prepared for press is almost completely preserved; all that is missing are the title pages, the preface, postscript and paragraph 6 in chapter 20. The manuscript and the printed text differ in places, because three days before his death Rudolf Steiner still made numerous corrections and additions to the galley proofs. After Rudolf Steiner's death the editing and implementation of these corrections were taken care of by Dr Hilma Walter. Ita Wegman wrote a preface and a postscript. The book was published in September 1925. The proposed second and perhaps even third volume never appeared. To continue the work, Ita Wegman published various items in the supplement to the journal *Natura* for members of the Medical Section in 1926–31, based on suggestions and notes deriving from her work with Rudolf Steiner. She published further medical essays in the journal *Natura* itself between 1926 and 1932. These have been combined and published under the title *Im Anbruch des Wirkens für eine Erweiterung der Heilkunst nach geisteswissenschaftlicher Menschenkunde*, Arlesheim: Natura Verlag 1956.

Part of Rudolf Steiner's manuscript has been printed in facsimile in *Beiträge zur Rudolf Steiner Gesamtausgabe* Nr. 58/59, Dornach, Herbst 1977, S. 3–21.

Substantial editorial changes compared to the 1925 edition are the following (comparing to G. Adams' and partly E. A. Frommer's and J. Josephson's translations).

page	line	changes
Title page		The words 'Part One' that followed the title have been omitted since the 2nd edition.
Contents		The heading 'Contents' was followed by the subtitle 'Part One'. This has been omitted since the 3rd edition.
40	14	'haem' to replace 'haematin'
77	25	'protein synthesis' to replace 'protein (activities)'
111	5	'in the nettle' to replace 'in the influence of the nettle'
114	28	'after the process of digestion' to replace 'after metabolism' or 'after the (digestive) process'.
114	31	'Suitably processed' to replace 'properly combined and administered' or 'in an appropriate form'

Translator's note

This being a written work, with the proofs of the original German edition checked by Rudolf Steiner himself, it seemed important to adhere as closely as possible to the original text. This did not prove too difficult a task on the whole, as the sentences are generally short and positively succinct, thesis following thesis, as it were.

The division into sentences, with use of full stops and semicolons, has been followed exactly, as has the division into paragraphs, including the unusual method of subdividing a paragraph by having a dash between two sentences.

Some problems arose with consistency of terminology. An example is the following. Rudolf Steiner and Ita Wegman used four terms to cover separating, secretory and eliminatory processes, and it seemed important to be consistent in the use of four English terms to match these. Two of the German terms, used both as verbs and verbal nouns, are *absondern* and *aussondern* (used once only). As the simplex, *sondern*, relates well to the English 'sunder', these two have been translated as 'separate off' and 'separate out'. The other pair, *abscheiden* and *ausscheiden*, have the simplex *scheiden*, which is an older term for 'separate' (today largely superseded by *trennen*) still used especially in chemistry and medicine. Here I have used the standard present-day terms for *abscheiden*, 'to secrete', and *ausscheiden*, 'to eliminate'. Maintaining this consistency has not always been easy. The terms would work well at times, but could also be problematical (see title of chapter 12!).

Translating decisions were taken in full recognition of the fundamental and germinal nature of this work.

Surbiton, July 1996   Anna Meuss

Further Reading

Rudolf Steiner:

Knowledge of the Higher Worlds (London: Rudolf Steiner Press).
Also published as *How to Know Higher Worlds* (New York:
Anthroposophic Press)
Occult Science (London: Rudolf Steiner Press)
The Philosophy of Spiritual Activity (London: Rudolf Steiner Press).
Also published as *Intuitive Thinking as a Spiritual Path* (New
York: Anthroposophic Press)
Theosophy (New York: Anthroposophic Press)

Other Authors:

A.I.D.S., The Deadly Seed, K. Dumke (London: Rudolf Steiner
Press)
The Anthroposophical Approach to Medicine (3 vols), F. Husemann
& O. Wolff (New York: Anthroposophic Press)
Anthroposophical Medicine, M. Evans & I. Rodger (London:
Thorsons)
Caring for the Sick at Home, T. v Bentheim et al (Edinburgh: Floris
Books)
Fundamentals of Artistic Therapy, M. Hauschka (London: Rudolf
Steiner Press)
A Guide to Child Health, M. Glöckler & W. Goebel (Edinburgh:
Floris Books)
In Place of the Self, How Drugs Work, R. Dunselman (Stroud:
Hawthorn Press)
Man on the Threshold, B. Lievegoed (Stroud: Hawthorn Press)
Phases, B. Lievegoed (London: Rudolf Steiner Press)
Rhythmical Massage, M. Hauschka (London: Rudolf Steiner Press)
Rock Bottom, Beyond Drug Addiction, ARTA (Stroud: Hawthorn
Press)

Other information

In-Patient Facilities
In-patient facilities exist in Austria, Germany, Italy, Netherlands, Sweden and Switzerland, ranging from university teaching hospitals to nursing homes and facilities for rehabilitation of drug addiction.

In the English-speaking world there exist the following centres:

(General medicine and psychiatry)
Park Attwood Clinic
Trimpley, Bewdley
Worcestershire
DY12 1RE
England

(Anthroposophically oriented rehabilitation centre and nursing home)
Raphael Medical Centre
Hollanden Park
Coldharbour Lane
Hildenborough
Tonbridge, Kent
TN11 9LE
England

Out-Patient Facilities
Details of anthroposophical medical practitioners may be obtained from the professional associations of anthroposophical doctors. (See list under professional associations.)

Manufacturers and Distributors of Anthroposophical Medicines
Weleda and also Wala have representations worldwide. Head offices:

Abnoba Heilmittel GmbH
Hohenzollernstrasse 16
D-75177-Pforzheim
Germany

Novipharm GmbH
Klagenfurderstrasse 164
A-9210-Pörtschach
Austria

Helixor Heilmittel GmbH
Postfach 8
D-7463-Rosenfeld 1
Germany

Wala Heilmittel GmbH
D-7325-Eckwälden/Bad Boll
Germany

Weleda AG
CH-4144-Arlesheim
Switzerland

Professional Associations and Trainings:
There are professional organisations, training facilities and courses for doctors, nurses, art therapists, eurythmy therapists, rhythmical masseurs and others. In the English-speaking world the following medical associations can be contacted:

Australia
Australian Anthroposophical Medical Association inc.
4 Hamilton Parade
Pymble 2073, NSW

Canada
Canadian Association for Anthroposophic Medicine
PO Box 335
Thornhill
Ontario, L3T 4A2

New Zealand
New Zealand Association of Anthroposophical Doctors
11 Woodford Road
Mt Eden
Auckland

South Africa
Anthroposophical Medical Association of Southern Africa
6 Crescent Road
Wynberg 7800 Cape

United Kingdom
Anthroposophical Medical Association
c/o Park Attwood Clinic
nr. Bewdley
Worcs, DY12 1RE

USA
Physicians Association for Anthroposophical Medicine
PO Box 269
Kimberton, PA 19442

Member Associations of the International Federation of Anthroposophical Medical Associations IVAA also exist in most European countries, as well as in Peru, Brazil and Argentina.

For further information contact the worldwide centre for the anthroposophical medical movement:

The Medical Section
School for Spiritual Science
Goetheanum
CH-4143 Dornach
Switzerland